Brilliantly combines the wisdom of Judaism and the forms and meanings of the Hebrew letters in an easy-to-use introduction to hatha yoga techniques.

Can yoga be *Jewish?* Yes! By blending traditional hatha yoga postures and the forms of the Hebrew *aleph-bet*, yoga teacher Steven Rapp shows how you can use this ancient health practice to deepen your Jewish spirituality.

Aleph-Bet Yoga shows us how to:

- Integrate the meaning of each Hebrew letter with the common name of the corresponding hatha yoga pose.

- Connect all twenty-seven Hebrew letters with hatha yoga poses that correspond to the shapes of the letters.

- Weave together the meaning of each Hebrew letter with the Sanskrit word for the yoga pose and a biblical phrase in meditation.

"The real miracle is in how the poses affect the mind and the heart. An increase in flexibility in the mind and heart is a gift that benefits all who come in contact with us. The false division of the human being as body, mind, and spirit are extinguished and we become whole. This gift of wholeness is a result of sustained organized practice. The blessing is in the effort itself, the results in the hands of the Creator."

—**Hart Lazer,** yoga teacher

"Founded on universal social and moral principles, yoga is adopted by people of all religions…. Steven Rapp's contribution is welcome, if it encourages even more to practice yoga, and thereby develop their physical, mental, spiritual and religious well-being."

—**Shyam Mehta,** co-author of *Yoga: The Iyengar Way*

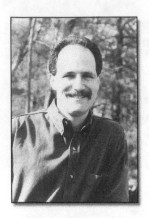

Steven A. Rapp has been a yoga practitioner for over ten years and is a yoga teacher in Boston. He also teaches religious school at Temple Beth David in Canton, Massachusetts, and offers personal instruction to those seeking to link traditional yoga practice and Judaism. He lives with his wife and three children in Randolph, Massachusetts.

"*Aleph-Bet Yoga* provides a form of movement that prepares the body for the work of *tikkun olam,* repairing the world. By putting our bodies into optimal condition with yoga while creating a Jewish focus and intent with Hebrew letters, I believe that we can act more effectively to make the world a better place."

— from Chapter 1

"We are now recovering an ancient sense of unity of body and soul. Steven A. Rapp is one of the pioneers in this area, working in the modality of yoga merged with the ancient practice of meditating on the Hebrew letters, the instruments of the divine act of creating the universe."

—Tamar Frankiel, Ph.D., and Judy Greenfeld, co-authors of *Entering the Temple of Dreams: Jewish Prayers, Movements, and Meditations for the End of the Day* and *Minding the Temple of the Soul: Balancing Body, Mind, and Spirit through Traditional Jewish Prayer, Movement, and Meditation*

"*Aleph-Bet Yoga* teaches us that when soul, body, and mind come together the journey toward understanding and wholeness is ever greater."

—Karyn D. Kedar, author of *The Dance of the Dolphin: Finding Prayer, Perspective and Meaning in the Stories of Our Lives*

JEWISH LIGHTS Publishing

Sunset Farm Offices, Route 4, P.O. Box 237
Woodstock, VT 05091
Tel: (802) 457-4000   Fax: (802) 457-4004

www.jewishlights.com
Find us on Facebook®
Facebook is a registered
trademark of Facebook, Inc.

COVER DESIGN: LYNNE WALKER

Aleph-Bet
YOGA

Embodying the Hebrew Letters for
Physical and Spiritual Well-Being

Steven A. Rapp

Foreword by Tamar Frankiel, Ph.D., and Judy Greenfeld
Preface by Hart Lazer

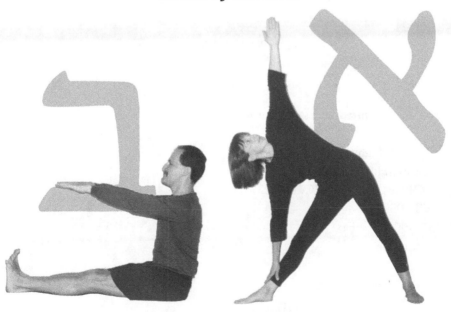

JEWISH LIGHTS Publishing
Woodstock, Vermont

Aleph-Bet Yoga:
Embodying the Hebrew Letters for Physical and Spiritual Well-Being

2012 Quality Paperback Edition, Second Printing

Library of Congress Cataloging-in-Publication Data
Rapp, Steven A., 1964–
   Aleph-bet yoga : embodying the Hebrew letters for physical and spiritual well-being / Steven A. Rapp.
        p.   cm.
   Includes bibliographical references.
   ISBN 1-58023-162-4
   1. Yoga, Haṭha. 2. Spiritual life—Judaism. 3. Hebrew language—Alphabet—Religious aspects—Judaism.   I. Title.
   RA781.7 .R37 2001
   613.7'046—dc21

                                              2001006126

10   9   8   7   6   5   4   3   2

Manufactured in the United States of America

Published by Jewish Lights Publishing
A Division of LongHill Partners, Inc.
Sunset Farm Offices, Route 4, P.O. Box 237
Woodstock, VT 05091
Tel: (802) 457-4000   Fax: (802) 457-4004
www.jewishlights.com

For my wife, **Ulrike,** and our children,
Hannah, Joshua, and **Rebecca**—
living proof that miracles do happen.

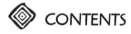 CONTENTS

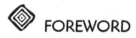 FOREWORD

by Tamar Frankiel and Judy Greenfeld

Physical discipline and textual study—together? Ten years ago this was a new concept, so radical that we were often challenged as we spoke to Jewish groups around the country: Judaism doesn't have any tradition of exercise, does it? Nobody does movement when they're praying! Yoga for Jews? Tai chi for Jews? Whoever heard of such a thing?

While it is true that Judaism (and, for that matter, other major Western religions) never developed a system of body disciplines connected to spiritual work like those of Asian cultures, the Rabbis were concerned about health of the body. Many were specifically involved in working with the body, either as official physicians or as healers within the folk tradition. In the nineteenth century, as the population became more confined and more sedentary, some rabbis began emphasizing the need for exercise. Most emphatically, they saw the body as a temple—a microcosm of the lost Holy Temple in Jerusalem, and thus a mirror of God's Temple that existed in the heavenly dimensions.

Now, many more people have accepted the idea of holiness of the body. We are recovering an ancient sense of unity of body and soul. These ideas are emerging as part of a collective development in what might be called "collective consciousness." Those who work with the body have become more and more willing to integrate spiritual approaches to alignment and healing; and people attracted to spiritual work look for a physical correlate for their work. Within a Jewish framework, more physical disciplines are able to combine their work with Jewish insights. Steven A. Rapp is one of the pioneers in this area, working in the modality of yoga merged with the ancient practice of meditating on the Hebrew letters, the instruments of the divine act of creating the universe.

We are delighted to see this work: first, as confirmation that interest in the body is not just a fad but a movement that is being enriched and developed as each practitioner puts his or her work before a larger audience. Second, hatha yoga itself is known in the East and West as one of the great tools of healing because of the flexibility and stimulation it provides for all areas of the body. Steven Rapp is to be congratulated for making this method available to Jews who may have avoided yoga because of its associations with another religion. Third, the focus on Hebrew letters helps strengthen our connections to our ancient tongue, our interest in the language itself, and, eventually, our desire to learn more deeply the words of our ancestors.

Finally, yoga brings into the physical realm an important aspect of every spiritual tradition. The connotation of the word is to attach or concentrate one's attention. Etymologically, *yoga* is related to our word *yoke,* that which brings the energies of the "animal" under control. In Jewish spiritual practice, we are talking about *kavannah,* or the ability to "aim" one's mind—and body—at a target. This discipline of physical and mental self-control is invaluable, whatever one's other spiritual inclinations. Practiced within the forms of Hebrew letters, it will take on new life.

Invigorating the life of the body will, as Rabbi Abraham Isaac Kook argued in 1920, enliven the entire Jewish people. As we have shown in our own work, our prayer life will become more meaningful and more dynamic. Our energy for daily work will increase. Our sensitivity to our own feelings and those of others will be enhanced. Our work as a "priestly" people will develop in ways we have not yet imagined.

—Tamar Frankiel and Judy Greenfeld

Tamar Frankiel and Judy Greenfeld are co-authors of *Minding the Temple of the Soul: Balancing Body, Mind, and Spirit through Traditional Jewish Prayer, Movement, and Meditation* and *Entering the Temple of Dreams: Jewish Prayers, Movements, and Meditations for the End of the Day* (both Jewish Lights, 1997 and 2000); Tamar is also author of *The Gift of Kabbalah: Discovering the Secrets of Heaven, Renewing Your Life on Earth* (Jewish Lights, 2001).

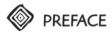 PREFACE

by Hart Lazer

Why Practice?

We expend energy in many ways. We talk with our friends and loved ones, go to work, hurry from place to place, from task to task, with little time left to feel and respond to our bodies and our beings as a whole. Consequently we often operate out of reflex conditioning or feelings of duty and responsibility. This overloading tends to manifest itself as resentments and frustrations that lead us to act in ways that don't originate from the core of our being. Without regularly nurturing and taking the time to honor that core we become alienated from it.

The techniques that best allow us to gain access to our core self vary from person to person. Whatever method we use must penetrate through our psychological and emotional layers to a quieter place within, a place of silence that effortlessly generates healing and nurturing. A well-organized yoga practice will bring us to that place.

About five years ago I was approached by Rabbi David A. Cooper to help bring yoga postures into the Jewish retreat setting. As a practicing yoga student, teacher, and observant Jew, I had often asked myself, "How does one remain a good Jew and still practice yoga in a deep way?" I had often viewed Judaism's neglect of the physical body at the expense of intellectual pursuits as a fundamental weakness in traditional Judaism. Yet in the western world, until just recently, the false division of the human body into either physical, mental, and spiritual has been all-pervasive. How then does one practice yoga and Judaism without selling out either side?

For me it came through recognition that yoga has the technology and makes the technology available for each of us to become a more virtuous person. To practice yoga we need not change our religious beliefs. In fact, yoga philosophy developed in a culture and time in which the notion of religion did not imply one group versus another. Rather it was designed to teach one how to live a virtuous life. Thus many people who were already practicing in some religion found yoga to expand their capacity to worship as well as to bring more happiness and fullness to their lives.

As shown by author Steven Rapp in *Aleph-Bet Yoga*, and throughout hatha yoga literature in general, the discovery of self is done through the concreteness of the body. When Rabbi Cooper first suggested bringing the yoga postures and the Hebrew alphabet together—a concept that Steven Rapp has expanded upon in his Aleph-Bet Yoga series—I tried it with some friends. We looked at the Hebrew letters and then found poses that were close in shape to the *otiyot*. We then practiced recalling B. K. S. Iyengar's comment that the body is a temple and the *asanas* are the prayers.

Yoga practice *is* much like prayer. It is the communion of body, mind, and spirit. The peaceful state brought about by yoga practice is often experienced as a cessation of chronological time along with a recognition that there is no difference between us and any other living being. We are no longer Jews or Christians or Muslims; we just are.

Asanas and *pranayamas,* the exercises Rapp guides us through in this book, are two of the eight limbs of yoga that focus on the physical being. To a large extent they are the parts of the eight-fold path that require discipline, intention, and motivation. There will be times in your practice session when you will want to laugh, cry, scream, and perhaps even throw this book across the room. Feel free to do all of these, then pick up the book and begin the poses again.

Along with improved discipline, one will also experience through regular yoga practice the physical and mental benefits that the postures offer: increased strength, stamina, and flexibility; the toning of muscles, ligaments, and nerves; enhanced capacities for concentration and relaxation. However, the real miracle is in how the poses affect the mind and the heart. An increase of flexibility in the mind and the heart is a gift that benefits all who come in contact with us. The false division of the human being as a body, mind, and spirit are extinguished and we become whole. This gift of wholeness is a result of sustained organized practice. The blessing is in the effort itself, the results in the hands of the Creator.

May the practice of yoga bring you great joy.

—Hart Lazer

Hart Lazer is a popular yoga teacher in Manitoba, Canada. His work and techniques were one of the inspirations behind David A. Cooper's book *Renewing Your Soul: A Guided Retreat for the Sabbath and Other Days of Rest,* which was revised and reissued as *The Handbook of Jewish Meditation Practices: A Guide for Enriching the Sabbath and Other Days of Your Life* (Jewish Lights, 2000).

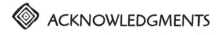 ACKNOWLEDGMENTS

I would like to thank all those who helped make this project possible, particularly my family and the influential teachers I have had. First, I thank my wife, Ulrike, for suggestions, for moral support, and for posing so beautifully for the photos in this book. I thank my children—Hannah, Joshua, and Rebecca—for their help with the original concept and for practicing the letter poses with me. Next, I want to thank my father, Peter Rapp, for taking the photographs in this book and for staying up late writing term papers with me years ago. Thanks to my mother, Anita Rapp (of blessed memory), for teaching me to look for the meaning of words. I also want to thank my stepmother, Esta Rapp, for sending me on my first trip to Israel—a trip that changed my view of all things Jewish forever.

Thanks to all my yoga teachers, including Nanda Rao of Arlington, Virginia, and Ricki Middleton of the Lotus Yoga Center in Silver Spring, Maryland, for my first yoga lessons, patience, and smiles. Also, thanks to Elizabeth Robboy of Somerville, Massachusetts, for her example and encouragement. A special thanks to B. K. S. Iyengar for his light and wisdom that has reached me through his students and his writings.

A deep thanks *(toda raba)* to Rabbi Daniel Judson of Temple Beth David of the South Shore in Canton, Massachusetts, for his inspiration and open mind in helping me shape this project. Thanks to Rabbi Lawrence Kushner for the inspiration I received from his many books. I also thank the people of Kibbutz Heftzi-Bah for helping me to learn Hebrew and for introducing me to my wife.

I would also like to thank Hart Lazer, whose connection of the Hebrew letters to hatha yoga *asanas* helped inspire this book, and Rabbi David A. Cooper, who brought Lazer's work to my attention in his book *Renewing Your Soul: A Guided Retreat for the Sabbath and Other Days of Rest.*

Thanks to Donald Nelson, for introducing me to poetry writing, and to poets Philip Levine and Jane Shore, for their instruction and encouragement while I was at Tufts University. Thanks to William Carlos Williams, for the influence his poems have had on my poetry and for his example as both a poet and a man of science.

Finally, I would like to thank all the people at Jewish Lights for helping bring this project to print. First, thanks to author Nancy Sohn Swartz, for introducing me to Jewish Lights. Next, thanks to Stuart M. Matlins, the publisher of Jewish Lights, for his vision and support of this unique project. Thanks to managing editor Emily Wichland, for her patience and guidance throughout the process. A special thanks to editor Donna Zerner, for her invaluable insights and feedback. Thanks to all who helped with the design and production of the book.

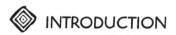 INTRODUCTION

Yoga has changed me in many positive ways: physically, mentally, and spiritually. Over the past twelve years it has helped me survive the stresses of full-time work, parenting, and life in our busy society. Yoga has helped me counteract the stiffening effects of the long hours I spend in chairs as a sedentary office worker. Yoga has helped me keep my balance during the periods of extreme stress and sleep deprivation known to all parents. And generally, it has helped me tap an otherwise hidden reservoir of energy within me so that I can offer my best to the world and those I love.

As a Jewish adult I find that yoga has helped me open my spiritual and intuitive channels, giving me an increased sense of awe in everyday surroundings. Yoga has provided me with a sense of presence in my relationships with people and in my experience of God. In this way, yoga has given me a deeper awareness of my purpose in this world. As a Jewish person I have always wanted to give my yoga practice an explicitly Jewish context. By focusing on the Hebrew letters when I practice yoga, I feel present before God as a full person—body and spirit.

Aleph-Bet Yoga is an introduction to yoga through a Jewish perspective. *Aleph-Bet Yoga* is unique because it is also about learning to use the whole self—body, mind, and spirit—to relate to Judaism. Using words in poetry, photos, and instructional text, *Aleph-Bet Yoga* provides a uniquely Jewish context for practicing hatha yoga. But *Aleph-Bet Yoga* is not just for Jewish people. I have led numerous Aleph-Bet Yoga sessions for people of all ages and backgrounds. I have seen firsthand the tremendously positive response people have to yoga combined with the Hebrew letters, regardless of their religious background.

East Meets West

As a Peace Corps volunteer in Benin, West Africa, I had a Muslim friend, Ibrahim, who saw me practicing Hebrew calligraphy one day. With a big smile, he asked me to teach him the Hebrew letters—"the language of Moses!" he said. I agreed, provided that he teach me to write the letters of Arabic.

Over the next few months, after morning coffee and bread, Ibrahim and I would sit down to draw letters and words while discussing the similarities of the Bible and the Koran. I learned to appreciate the underlying similarities of seemingly disparate cultures as we sat side by side, penning the flowing characters of the languages used by the children of Abraham.

In the years since leaving West Africa, I have continued to envision and experiment with ways of synthesizing seemingly opposing or unrelated viewpoints. I have looked for similarities among peoples and cultures, even where they appear superficially disconnected. I believe that our underlying human nature connects us all. I believe that there is an abundance of common ground.

In the book *Honey from the Rock: An Introduction to Jewish Mysticism* (Jewish Lights, 2000), Rabbi Lawrence Kushner says that "The Jewish response to the holy comes historically from the juncture of East and West. It is a system eternally bent on synthesizing the two."[1] *Aleph-Bet Yoga* is my attempt at synthesizing elements of East and West through a Jewish context, using words in poetry and movements of the human body. It is my attempt at combining my interests in Judaism and hatha yoga. It is my attempt at bringing Western bodies and minds together after centuries of alienation. And in a small way, it is my attempt at finding common ground between the Indian and Jewish peoples, who, because of the geopolitics of the twentieth century, found themselves on different sides of the Cold War.

Hebrew Letters Come Alive

A few years ago, Rabbi Gedalia Druin, a *sofer* (Torah scribe), came to Temple Beth David of the South Shore in Canton, Massachusetts, to repair one of the synagogue's Torah scrolls. Rabbi Druin invited students of the Sunday school to watch him finish his work on the scroll. It was an experience that dramatically changed my view of the Hebrew *aleph-bet*.

Before Rabbi Druin started, he invited the youngest children of the school into the social hall, where he was working. He asked for volunteers and proceeded to pose them as various Hebrew letters. He explained that the letters were not just marks of ink on a page (or scroll). Rather, each letter was a representation of something. Some letters gave a hint of their origin, like *yud*, which looks like a hand, or *yad* in Hebrew. He explained that each word was really a series of pictures ordered in a special way.

That day, I realized that there were many ways to teach Hebrew and Torah, using our bodies, not just our minds. I saw that we could relate to the letters physically as well as intellectually. And I realized that a physical connection to the *aleph-bet* could strengthen our attempts to learn the letters and their sounds.

As Easy as *Aleph, Bet, Gimmel...*

Aleph-Bet Yoga is aimed at a wide range of audiences, from children learning their *aleph-bet* in religious school, to adults who are familiar with hatha yoga or other forms of meditation but would like their practice to have a Jewish context, to people of all ages who care about their health and are curious about yoga but have not known where to begin.

If you are curious about hatha yoga, *Aleph-Bet Yoga* provides a safe introduction to the basic hatha yoga postures and techniques. It will orient you, get you going on the basics, and show you where to go for more depth. If you are one of the tens of thousands of Jews who already practice hatha yoga, *Aleph-Bet Yoga* will connect your yoga with something explicitly Jewish. With its Jewish content and intent, *Aleph-Bet Yoga* will enhance rather than interfere with your religious identity. If you are interested in a Jewish alternative for improving and maintaining good health and well-being, practicing Aleph-Bet Yoga will provide you with many of the health benefits that yoga has to offer. Finally, if you are interested in letters becoming words—poetry and language—*Aleph-Bet Yoga* will introduce you to intriguing phrases and to twenty-nine original poems.

At the end of the book is a list of resources that contains the names, addresses, and/or web addresses that can connect you with yoga teachers in your area. It also contains the names of other printed matter and videotapes that can help you deepen your Judaism or your yoga. Good luck!

1 ◈ What Is Aleph-Bet Yoga?

The Body Connection

One difference between the major religions of the East and those of the West is the role of the human body. In many of the Eastern religions, such as Hinduism, Taoism, and Buddhism, the body is considered part of the whole self, a temple of the soul. Many of the Eastern religions include specific exercises for strengthening and purifying both body and mind. Generally, however, the major Western religions, such as Judaism and Christianity, do not explicitly discuss methods for exercising and caring for the human body. Rather, the major Western religions, particularly Judaism, have tended to emphasize and idealize intellectual prowess.

But if we look closely at the Jewish texts, we can find acknowledgment of the human body's implicit holiness. In Genesis, the Torah tells us that we (bodies and minds) were created in God's image. Furthermore, Deuteronomy tells us to "choose life" (30:19). This commandment can be taken as an admonishment to take care of our bodies rather than giving in to our inclinations that might hurt us.

Several Jewish prayers also express the inherent sacredness of the body, emphasizing the importance of a healthy body in leading a full life. For example, the prayer that begins with *modeh ani* (literally, "I thank you") is a prayer one says to thank God for restoring the soul to the body upon waking up. This is clear recognition that without body and soul united, we can serve no purpose; we cannot study, we cannot pray, we cannot do good deeds. So we give thanks for the chance each day to move forward with body and mind.

Similarly, the prayer known as the *Asher yatzar* (literally, "who has formed") has an obvious focus on the body. It is a prayer that gives thanks to God for forming the human body with wisdom. It is traditionally said after one goes to the bathroom in the morning. It is a humble acknowledgment that if the body did not work according to its divine design—for example, if one of the openings were closed when it should be open, or one of the cavities in our organs were open when it should be closed—"we would be unable to stay alive and stand before You."

The *V'ahavta* prayer commands you to "love your God with all your heart, with all your soul, and with all your strength." Here again, we find recognition that we need more than just intellect to fulfill ourselves as Jews. In the same way, in the *Mishehberach* prayer, we ask God, as the source of strength, to heal our bodies so that we can make the world a better place. In both of these prayers, we see that in order to participate fully in the drama of existence, we must be healthy and strong in body as well as in spirit.

In the Torah commentary known as the Talmud, there is a parable of the King's Garden. In the story, the king hired a blind man and a lame man to guard his orchard, thinking that neither would be able to steal his fruit, but together they could guard his property. One day, they realized that by combining their abilities they could indeed reach the fruit on the trees. The lesson of the parable is not how to steal fruit but rather that our minds and bodies are not separate beings. Without the mind, our body is like the blind man, unable to find our way or see the fruit. Without a healthy body, we are like the lame man, unable to fulfill the mind's intentions or reach the fruit hanging above our heads.

Can Yoga Be Jewish?

Traditionally, Judaism has not included an explicit and detailed physical wellness component as some of the Eastern philosophical traditions have. For example, tai chi, a mixture of dance and martial arts, is recognized as the physical complement of the intellectual and spiritual components of Buddhism, Confucianism, and Taoism. While there is no separate body of traditional Jewish instructions for wellness, any health-centered behavior that helps us to fulfill the *mitzvah* of "choosing life" could be viewed as Jewish in its intent. If we practice yoga postures and our intention is focused on the Hebrew letters and their meanings, it could be viewed as "Jewish yoga."

Historically, mainstream Judaism's lack of a body component was largely a reaction to the ancient Greek idolization of the human body. In the times of the Hellenistic Greek empire, many Jews refused to participate in any part of Greek culture because it was seen as opposed to the monotheistic philosophy of Judaism. They refused to speak Greek, eat Greek foods, or participate in Greek sports or leisure activities, which were all part of the pagan religious system. As a result, Jewish culture discouraged any activities that focused solely on improving the human body.

Later, in the Diaspora, this thinking was reinforced by the way the rabbis taught Jews to connect with God in the absence of the Temple and by centuries of landlessness. In many countries and cultures around the world, Jews were not allowed to own land. With no land to cultivate or defend by arms, and with prayer and study as the ways to hear God's voice in one's life, Jewish culture generally emphasized and idealized intellectual skills over physical fitness.

Quite a contrast to today, when most Jews, particularly of the baby boom generation and later, feel no threat to their Jewish identities when they speak the local language, eat the local cuisine, or exercise at the gymnasium. In fact, with our current knowledge of science and medicine, many Jews today have a holistic approach to their well-being and an interest in keeping their bodies healthy along with their minds, emotions, and spirits. This may explain why so many Jews are drawn to yoga as an all-around wellness system that complements the rest of their Jewish lives.

A Jew in the Lotus Position

The sixties and seventies were a time when many great teachers came to America from India and the Far East. These men and women came here to introduce the Eastern perspective and teach the healing arts like yoga, tai chi, and meditation, but their positive efforts were blurred by the tumult of those times. As a result, many Americans were left with the idea that activities such as yoga and meditation have more to do with the counterculture, protesting the Vietnam War, and shocking one's parents than with good health and spiritual development.

Now, however, Americans are ready to give the Eastern methods a closer look. Alternative medicine is "respectable," and skyrocketing medical costs, insolvent health maintenance organizations, and soaring prescription drug costs have given us all economic incentives to look for health care possibilities other than pills and hospital procedures. In fact, many health insurance plans today support alternatives such as hatha yoga, tai chi, and meditation for their stress reduction potential. Imagine that in 1960!

In recent years, millions of Americans have begun to include hatha yoga in their exercise routines. It is offered at most fitness centers, gymnasiums, Jewish Community Centers, and the like. In some parts of the country, yoga classes are now as common as aerobics or kickboxing. But many people have begun to realize that yoga is more than just exercise. In fact, in addition to being a comprehensive preventative medicine for the body, yoga can be a profound source of spiritual and emotional well-being.

What Is Yoga?

The word *yoga* is derived from the Sanskrit root *yuj,* meaning to attach or to concentrate one's attention. It can also mean union or communion. In other words, yoga is the systematic methodology of joining all the powers of body, mind, and soul to God or Oneness.[2]

There are four main paths of yoga: the yoga of action, the yoga of devotion, the yoga of knowledge, and the yoga of physical and mental control. This last type of yoga is known as raja, or royal, yoga and is what most Westerners think of as yoga. In *Light on Yoga,* B. K. S. Iyengar describes the eight fundamental limbs, or stages, of this yoga:

1. Universal moral commandments
2. Self-purification by discipline
3. Posture
4. Rhythmic control of the breath
5. Withdrawal and emancipation of the mind from the domination of the senses and exterior objects
6. Concentration
7. Meditation
8. A state of super-consciousness brought about by profound meditation, in which the individual aspirant becomes one with the universal spirit[3]

Iyengar describes how, essentially, the eight branches aim to harmonize and integrate all aspects of the human being. The rules of personal conduct and moral principles are a social code, providing for harmony in personal relationships as well as in society at large. The postures are designed to harmonize the body in its surroundings and to maintain good physical health. Control of the breath and senses teaches control of the mind. And finally, concentration, meditation, and spiritual absorption harmonize the self with the Infinite. In this way, the eight branches form a practical philosophy that leads to increasingly deeper levels of physical and spiritual awareness and functioning, ultimately resulting in enlightenment.

Many Westerners are familiar with the specific branch of raja yoga called hatha yoga. Hatha yoga teaches mastery of the body and control of the breath. The word *hatha* means "force." It is derived from two roots: *ha,* the sun, and *tha,* the moon. Learning hatha yoga, therefore, is like learning to harmonize the active, fiery forces with the cooler, contemplative forces that are contained within us all. Hatha yoga uses poses, or *asanas,* that often mimic animals or forces found in the natural world to exercise and massage all parts of the body. Some of the basic hatha yoga movements are similar to the stretching exercises used by athletes all around the world.

Although hatha yoga is primarily a system of movements that tone the whole body, the contemplative movements also focus the mind for spiritual or meditative endeavors. While it can be practiced as a form of physical exercise, hatha yoga can be much more if practiced with the proper intention. Hatha yoga helps provide focus and balance, allowing people to apply themselves fully to all other facets of life.

In many ways, yoga provides the essential tools for not only surviving but thriving in our modern age. It is a means to bring the physical, mental, and emotional stresses of life under control. A regular yoga practice creates a feeling of overall well-being in many ways. It helps one regain lost flexibility, improve posture, and lessen or eliminate minor aches and pains. Yoga helps counteract the effects of long hours of office work spent in chairs, and the muscle stiffness and soreness that often accompany manual labor. The postures of yoga massage the internal organs and glandular systems, helping regulate the hormones, appetite, and blood circulation. Yoga increases the blood flow to the brain, improving concentration and memory. Yoga helps us let go of physical and emotional tension, deepens self-awareness, and increases intuition. In its meditative movements and breathing exercises, yoga cultivates calmness, which helps us modulate our emotions and increases compassion.

If we are out of balance physically, emotionally, or spiritually, we cannot reach our potential as human beings. But more than just helping us control the stresses that confront us, yoga cultivates the strength and the stillness within us that allow us to be fulfilled amidst the growing emptiness of our age. While yoga does not offer magical cures for illness, loneliness, or selfishness, it does provide the tools for understanding and improving ourselves in all aspects of our lives.

Is Yoga a Religion?

In *Light on Yoga*, Iyengar states clearly that "Yoga is not a religion by itself. It is the science of religions, the study of which will enable a *sadhaka* (aspirant) to better appreciate his own faith."[4] In the more than twelve years that I have been learning about and practicing yoga, many other yoga teachers have reaffirmed this conclusion. Hatha yoga is not a system of prayer, and practicing the *asanas,* or postures, does not conflict with one's personal religious beliefs. Rather, yoga complements a person's faith system by energizing the body and making space in one's mind for focusing personal thoughts and prayers.

Although Indian religious practices often intersect and overlap with yoga, yoga is not considered a religion for a variety of reasons. Yoga does not have a uniform set of beliefs, rituals, or requirements. Yoga does not have a single set of obligations of the kind that are normally associated with a religion, such as how often and where to pray.

Perhaps what confuses people about yoga and religion is that there are places in the West where yoga is taught that include a variety of Indian religious customs, chants, and prayers, usually at the start and finish of a class. Participation in such ritual, however, is not necessary for experiencing the positive results of yoga. Yoga that is taught in this manner is an expression of a particular teacher's set of beliefs or lineage. Such expression can be very important to the teacher, especially a teacher from India, and perhaps to some of the students. Usually it is done to create a positive atmosphere in which the yoga is effective for those particular participants. But students attend yoga classes voluntarily, and if they are uncomfortable with a form of religious expression practiced there, they have several choices. They may either choose not to participate in that portion of the class or substitute the chants or prayers with prayers of their own faith. Alternatively, students may look for a different class where no rituals or prayers are expressed.

On the other hand, outside the yoga studio, many people find that yoga practice brings a whole new mindfulness to their personal religious practice or spiritual endeavors. In Judaism, Jews are supposed to have proper *kavannah,* or intention, both in their prayers and in their actions to fulfill the *mitzvot,* or God's commandments. As yoga increases self-awareness, it helps many Jews to be conscious in their decisions and be present in their actions, thereby increasing their *kavannah.* Many people find that yoga also opens their intuitive channels, making them more receptive to subtle spiritual experiences that some might describe as an increased sense of awe. Through yoga, many grow to appreciate more fully the ceremonies and rituals of their own religious backgrounds.

What Is Aleph-Bet Yoga?

Aleph-Bet Yoga is a bridge between the physical and intellectual aspects of Judaism. It provides a method of moving our bodies through the Hebrew *aleph-bet* while focusing on the inner meanings of those letters. In this way, Aleph-Bet Yoga allows us to use our whole selves—body and mind—to relate to the Hebrew language and Judaism, and to feel connected to the letters and the language in a holistic way that simply reading or writing cannot achieve.

At the same time, *Aleph-Bet Yoga* uses words in poetry, photos, and symbols to provide a Jewish intention to the physical effort of caring for our bodies through hatha yoga.

Throughout Jewish history, the Hebrew alphabet has always been considered to have many levels of meaning. In *The Book of Letters: A Mystical Hebrew Alphabet* (Jewish Lights, 1990), Rabbi Lawrence Kushner describes how historically the Hebrew letters, the *otiyot*, have been a source of wisdom, meditation, and fantasy.[5] In the Jewish mystical tradition, the Hebrew letters are considered the divine instruments of God's energy, holy vessels carrying the light of God. For centuries, mystics have read, written, and meditated on the letters in ways that they hoped would bring them closer to the Divine.

Today, there is a remarkable concurrence of Jewish teachings that seek to integrate body movements with the Hebrew *aleph-bet*. Around the United States and in Israel, many people have been creatively integrating the movements of yoga, dance, and tai chi with the forms of the Hebrew letters. Some believe that the current generations of Jews are recreating some of the hidden mystical tradition that was lost in the Holocaust. Others feel that it is an organic return to our ancient roots of dance and movement that may have existed during the times of King Solomon's Temple.

In his book *Renewing Your Soul: A Guided Retreat for the Sabbath and Other Days of Rest*, Rabbi David A. Cooper offers ideas for what he calls moving meditation. One moving meditation he suggests is a series of hatha yoga poses that approximate twenty-two of the Hebrew letters, a series developed by Hart Lazer. With each letter and yoga pose, Cooper also suggests a reflection on the word or concept traditionally associated with each Hebrew letter (e.g., the letter *dalet* is a doorway, or *delet* in Hebrew, and he suggests imagining that you are a doorway).[6]

Aleph-Bet Yoga expands on this Hebrew–yoga connection in several ways. First, *Aleph-Bet Yoga* integrates Rabbi Cooper's descriptions of the meaning of each Hebrew letter with the meaning of the Sanskrit word or common name that describes the corresponding yoga pose. Many yoga poses are known by several names in English; for example, the "rooster" may in some places be referred to as a variation on the "mountain" pose. *Aleph-Bet Yoga* uses English translations that are common in American yoga classes and manuals.

Next, for each of the Hebrew letters, *Aleph-Bet Yoga* presents the letters formed into words—a poem I have written that weaves together the meaning of the letter, the name of the yoga pose, and a phrase containing the particular letter. The phrases come from a variety of Jewish sources: the Hebrew Bible, Hebrew prayers, and Jewish mystical writings. Through the poems and phrases, *Aleph-Bet Yoga* reaches beneath the superficial meanings of the English, Hebrew, and Sanskrit words and tries to find the place where East and West may have met long ago.

Finally, *Aleph-Bet Yoga* connects all of the twenty-seven Hebrew letters (i.e., the twenty-two regular Hebrew letters plus the five final letter symbols for *kaf, mem, nun, pey,* and *tzadi)* with hatha yoga poses that correspond to the shapes of the letters. *Aleph-Bet Yoga* also associates two of the Hebrew vowels, *kamatz* and *patach,* with two yoga poses that are important to do at the close of every yoga session.

Hatha yoga has hundreds of poses requiring varying levels of ability. *Aleph-Bet Yoga* presents poses that correspond (sometimes loosely) to the shape of the Hebrew letters while staying approachable at a beginner's level. Chapter 3 introduces the letters and yoga poses in the order of the Hebrew *aleph-bet* (i.e., in *aleph-*betical order). However, I do not recommend that you practice the poses in that order. Rather, in chapter 4, I have outlined a series of poses—what I call the Aleph-Bet Yoga series—that corresponds to the proper order of a yoga session.

The World Depends on Three Things

Aleph-Bet Yoga provides a form of movement that prepares the body for the work of *tikkun olam,* repairing the world. By putting our bodies into optimal condition with yoga while creating a Jewish focus and intent with the Hebrew letters, I believe that we can act more effectively to make the world a better place.

Although there may be differences between Eastern and Western customs, the fundamental values of societies are often the same. In *Light on Yoga,* Iyengar tells us that in the Hindu system, "the man who combines within his mortal frame knowledge, love, and selfless service is holy."[7] This is strikingly similar to the saying "*Al shlosha d'varim,*" found in the Jewish writings known as the *Pirkei Avot* ("Wisdom of Our Fathers") compiled in the second century C.E., which says that the world depends on three things: study, service (of God), and acts of lovingkindness.

Regardless of your background, I hope that the exercises and poems in the following chapters will stretch, strengthen, and energize you to study, serve, and perform many acts of lovingkindness. *Namaste.* Shalom. Salaam. Peace.

2 ◈ Getting Started with Hatha Yoga Poses

Where to Begin

There are a few simple guidelines you should follow when practicing hatha yoga poses.

Make Yourself at Home

Hatha yoga can be done just about anywhere, but the proper setting can allow you to get the most out of your practice. For example, a quiet, warm room with a 4-foot by 8-foot open space is best. Also, a hardwood floor or firm carpet gives your feet a good grip while you do the standing and balancing poses. A thin (quarter-inch) exercise mat, known in yoga circles as a sticky mat, works even better. But if a room with a soft carpet is the only space you can find, it will work just as well.

Try to choose a place where you will not be interrupted or distracted. Avoid direct sunlight; it is difficult to concentrate if the sun is in your eyes. You may choose to listen to soft music while practicing. Personally, I find it easier to "listen" to how my body feels in the poses when it is quiet. But some people find that music enhances their sense of focus and relaxation, and they enjoy their practice more with it.

Loosen Up

You should wear comfortable clothing while practicing yoga poses. Yoga can be done in street clothes, but gym shorts or sweatpants and a loose top work best. Belts, ties, and other restrictive clothing should be removed before you start. Also, yoga is best done without shoes or socks. Hatha yoga poses stretch the feet and ankles, and shoes or sneakers can restrict the movement. Socks can cause you to slip or slide, especially if you are on a smooth wooden floor.

Empty the Vessel

Your stomach and bladder should be empty before you begin. Yoga poses twist and massage your internal organs, and a full stomach or bladder can cause discomfort or nausea. This means that you should wait at least two hours after a big meal or one hour after a light meal or snack before practicing the poses. Similarly, you should go to the bathroom before starting. Many people do their yoga first thing in the morning or before going to sleep for this reason.

I find that the best time for my yoga practice is before a meal. Before breakfast, yoga gets the blood circulating in the body, and I am then more alert when I start my workday. Before lunch, my stomach is relatively empty, and I am not as stiff as I am first thing in the morning and not as tired as I am later in the day. Before dinner, I find yoga a great way to make a transition from the work day and relieve some of my stored tension.

Get an Attitude

While you practice the hatha yoga poses, it is important that you have a positive attitude. Try to smile in each pose. Smiling naturally relaxes the mind and body and will help you stretch better than if you are tight with a grimace or a frown. Even if you are feeling some discomfort in a pose, try to smile and relax into the stretch. Try to maintain a sense of humor. Remember that it will be a little bit easier each time you practice.

Breathe Deeply

Proper breathing is very important in hatha yoga. Basically, you should try to breathe evenly and deeply through the nose, not your mouth, when practicing a pose. Do not hold your breath. Use your whole lung capacity to breathe. Most of us use only the top third of our lungs when we breathe. While you practice yoga, it is important to inhale as deeply as you can, beginning by extending the diaphragm (the belly below the ribs), then the lower ribs, followed by the upper ribs. To exhale deeply, reverse the order, emptying the upper rib cage, lower rib cage, and diaphragm.

If you feel tightness in a muscle, do not fight it. Instead, use your breath to help you release the tension you feel. Inhale until you feel tightness, and then use your exhalation to push yourself gently and stretch a little deeper. Count your breaths for concentration—a full inhalation and exhalation constitute one breath. Hold each pose for three to five breaths (approximately 15 to 30 seconds). After you get the hang of counting breaths, you will find it easier than trying to keep an eye on the second hand of a clock.

Listen to Your Body

Pay attention to the signals you are getting from your body. The movements of hatha yoga should be done slowly and with care. Gently make adjustments to your body in each stretch. Do not bounce while stretching. Practicing in sight of a mirror can help you keep your spine, legs, and other parts of your body aligned.

Yoga can feel great, but it is normal to feel some discomfort when trying to stretch muscles and connective tissue that have not been stretched for many years (or ever). It is common to experience some unfamiliar physical sensations in some of the more challenging poses. Try to focus on your breathing instead of dwelling on discomfort or on your distance from the ideal pose. Try to concentrate on the shape of the Hebrew letter. Think of the divine energy in that shape. Focus on the meaning of the letter, the Hebrew phrase, or what the corresponding poem means to you.

If you experience sharp pain or excessive tightness, stop and do not continue in a pose. You should consult a physician before starting yoga if you have any preexisting injuries or conditions such as high blood pressure or arthritis, or if you could be pregnant. Also, consult a doctor if you feel pain in a joint rather than muscle aches after practicing hatha yoga.

Please do not be judgmental with yourself. Relax. Yoga is not an all-or-nothing activity. Do not be discouraged if you cannot finish the pose exactly as described during the first, the second, or even the twentieth time you try it. The precise forms will come with time. You will start to get the benefits of hatha yoga even as a beginner.

As you continue practicing the poses over time you may find that you experience some unexpected or uncomfortable emotions as well. These can range from unexpected laughter to anger or sadness. This is natural. Yoga increases our awareness of where in our bodies we are stuck physically, which can be related to emotional or psychological trauma, such as from an accident or injury. Notice the stuck spots, and use your breath to move through the resistance. Welcome any emotions and let them go. See this experience as part of the growth process.

Practice Regularly

As with any skill, the more you practice, the better you will get. And as with any skill, it is better to practice a little each day rather than once a week for a long time. Ideally, you should practice long enough to hold each pose for three to five breaths (approximately 15 to 30 seconds) and then rest between poses for 5 to 10 seconds. If you are just beginning, you might want to try the pose once, rest, and then try it again. For poses that stretch one side differently from the other, you should do the pose on one side, then the other. If time and your schedule permit, you should practice the poses every day for maximum benefit. As a start, however, twice a week for 30 minutes is probably manageable for most people. Try to find a day and time that works, and stick with it.

Proceed in an Orderly Fashion

Hatha yoga poses are grouped into categories. Generally, you should practice the poses of one category before moving on to the next. In most styles of hatha yoga, the poses are learned as a series of poses. *While the next chapter describes the hatha yoga poses in the order of the Hebrew aleph-bet, I do not recommend that you practice the poses in that order. Rather, in chapter 4, I have outlined a series of poses that would be appropriate for beginners.* If you do not have time to do the whole series, you may choose to focus on just a few letter poses. Alternatively, you may skip some poses that are similar within one of the categories, as noted in chapter 4.

Get a Little Class

I strongly recommend that while you are trying to learn about yoga through books and videos you take a regular (e.g., weekly) hatha yoga class at your nearest yoga center, Jewish Community Center, YMCA, fitness center, gym, or health care organization. There is no comparison between trying to teach yourself through reading and watching videos and having an experienced teacher who can guide and correct you.

Use Caution

Please keep in mind that although there are many health benefits from practicing yoga, it is always possible to injure yourself if you are not careful or if you do not follow the instructions correctly. The instructions contained in this book are designed for a beginner with average physical ability. ***If you have physical limitations, are pregnant, or have a preexisting injury or medical condition, use extra caution and consult with a physician before attempting the postures on your own.***

You should observe a few specific cautions as well. If you have high blood pressure, a detached retina, or an ear infection, you should avoid inverted poses like *urdhva prasarita padasana*, the pose associated with the letter *tzadi*. Inverted poses are also not recommended for women who are menstruating. For pregnant women, caution is advisable, although for most women all the poses are safe during the first trimester. After that, consult with your physician. If you suffer from a herniated or slipped disk, do not attempt the back-bending poses, including *urdhva dhanurasana* (final *pey*), *kapotasana (pey)*, *ustrasana (mem)*, *salabhasana I (shin)*, or *dhanurasana (samech)*. If you have ever injured your back, you should be extra careful with *ardha navasana (tet)* and *urdhva prasarita padasana (tzadi)* as well.

Where Do We Go from Here?

You may also want to consult the resource list at the end of the book. There is a list of names, addresses, and/or web addresses that can connect you with experienced yoga teachers in your area. It also contains the names of other printed matter and videotapes that can help you deepen your yoga or your Judaism.

3 ◈ Poses, Letters, and Words

The Proper Order of a Yoga Session

This chapter introduces the letters and yoga poses in the order of the Hebrew *aleph-bet* (i.e., in *aleph*betical order). However, as noted earlier, and as explained in more detail in chapter 4, I do not recommend that you practice the poses in that order. Rather, in chapter 4, "The Aleph-Bet Yoga Series—the Proper Order of a Yoga Session," I have outlined a series of poses that correlates to the best order for the poses.

Aleph

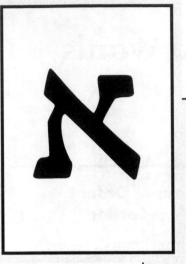

In Hebrew, this letter is a symbol for oxen. A corresponding yoga pose is *utthita trikonasana*, or the triangle pose.

בָּרוּךְ אַתָּה יְיָ אֱלֹהֵינוּ מֶלֶךְ הָעוֹלָם,
אֲשֶׁר יָצַר אֶת־הָאָדָם בְּחָכְמָה.

Bah-ruch ah-tah Ah-doh-nai, Eh-loh-hay-noo meh-lech hah-oh-lahm, ah-shehr yah-tsahr eht hah-ah-dahm b'choch-mah.

Blessed is God, Ruler of the universe, who has formed the human being with wisdom.

—from the daily prayer book

Body and spirit joined together
Like oxen yoked to work another day.
Like *ha*, the sun,
Yoked to *tha*, the moon.
Two triangles,
One ascending,
One descending,
To form a star.

Benefits: This standing pose stretches and strengthens feet, knees, and spine. Develops good posture.

1. Stand straight with feet together and arms by your sides. Inhale.

2. Exhale, walk or jump your feet apart 4 feet (as wide as the length of one of your legs), and raise your arms parallel to the floor, palms facing downward.

3. Keeping your hips facing forward, turn your right foot 90 degrees from the left so that the heel of your right foot is in line with the arch of your left foot.

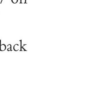

4. Inhale, and stand up as tall as you can. As you exhale, reach to the right as far as you can, with straight arms and straight legs, as if reaching for a rescue line and your feet are stuck to the floor. Without collapsing your rib cage, lower your straight right arm and hand to wherever it touches your right leg, and raise your straight left arm so that it is pointing straight up. Do not put pressure on your right hand/leg.

5. Inhale, turn your head, and try to look up at your left hand. If this feels like too much of a stretch for your neck, you can face forward.

6. Smile, and take three to five deep breaths (15 to 30 seconds), releasing any tension you feel in your hamstrings or lower back with each exhalation. You should feel your weight on the outer edges of your feet.

7. Inhale, reaching up toward the ceiling with your left hand. Bring your torso back to the center with your arms parallel to the floor.

8. Switch the position of your feet, and do steps 3 through 7 on the left side.

9. Jump or walk your feet back together, and bring your arms back down to your sides.

Bet

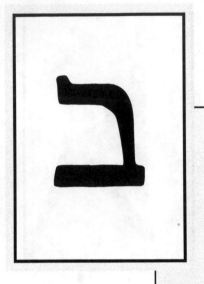

This letter is a symbol for a house. A corresponding yoga pose is a variation on *dandasana*, the stick pose, with arms extended.

אָהַבְתִּי מְעוֹן בֵּיתֶךָ,
וּמְקוֹם מִשְׁכַּן כְּבוֹדֶךָ.

Ah-hahv-tee m'ohn bay-teh-chah, oom-kohm meesh-kahn k'voh-deh-chah.

I love Your house and the dwelling place of Your glory.

—from the daily prayer book

The body is a house
Made of sticks and skin and soul,
An open tent
Where we dwell in God's glory,
Looking out to do good deeds.

Benefits: This seated pose stretches and strengthens feet, calves, thighs, lower back, shoulders, and arms. Improves seated posture. Strengthens and aligns the spine.

1. Sit on the floor with your legs together and extended straight out.

2. Flex your feet so that your toes point back toward your body.

3. Inhale, and sit up as straight as possible, lifting your rib cage, lifting your chin. Straighten your spine as if there were a string running through your spine and through your head, and someone were pulling it up.

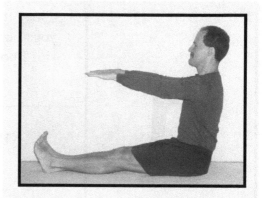

4. Exhale, and straighten your arms in front of you so that they are parallel to the floor. Reach straight ahead through your fingertips, but keep your back straight up and down.

5. Smile, and take three to five deep breaths.

6. Lower your arms. Shake your legs gently.

Gimmel

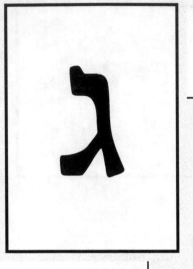

This letter is a symbol for a camel. A corresponding yoga pose is a variation of *virabhadrasana*, the warrior I pose.

עַל שְׁלֹשָׁה דְבָרִים הָעוֹלָם עוֹמֵד:
עַל הַתּוֹרָה, וְעַל הָעֲבוֹדָה,
וְעַל גְּמִילוּת חֲסָדִים.

Ahl sh'loh-shah deh-vah-reem hah-oh-lahm oh-mayd: ahl hah-toh-rah, v'ahl hah-ah-voh-dah, v'ahl geh-mee-loot chah-sah-deem.

The world depends on three things: study, service (of God), and acts of lovingkindness.

—*Pirkei Avot 2:3*

Like a camel,
I go forward
To carry goodness into the world.
Acts of love and kindness
Are my joyful burden.

Like a peaceful warrior,
I arm myself for repairing the world.
I must keep my body strong.
Acts of lovingkindness
Exercise my soul.

Benefits: This pose stretches and strengthens the groin muscles, knees, hips, spine, shoulders, and neck. Increases breathing. Warms body. Improves circulation.

1. Stand straight with feet together and arms by your sides. Inhale.

2. Exhale, and jump or walk your feet 4 feet apart with both feet pointing forward.

3. Inhale, raise your arms straight up in the air, and reach up as high as you can. Look up between your hands.

4. Turn the right foot 90 degrees so that your right heel is in line with the arch of your left foot.

5. While still stretching upward with your arms, exhale, and rotate your hips to face right (the same direction to which your right foot is pointing).

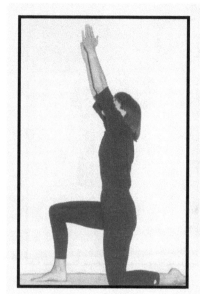

6. Bend your right knee 90 degrees, come onto the ball of your left foot, and drop your left knee to the floor. Or, for a deeper stretch, keep your left leg straight and your left foot flat on the floor.

7. Smile, and take three to five deep breaths.

8. Inhale, and straighten your legs. Rotate your hips back to center.

9. Exhale, and lower your arms.

10. Repeat steps 3 through 9 on the other side.

11. Jump your feet back together.

Dalet

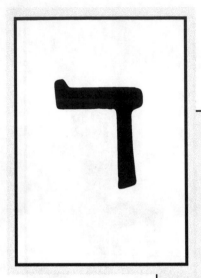

This letter is a symbol of a doorway. A corresponding yoga pose is a variation on *uttanasana*, the forward extension pose.

וַיִּשְׁכַּב שְׁמוּאֵל עַד־הַבֹּקֶר
וַיִּפְתַּח אֶת־דַּלְתוֹת בֵּית־יְהוָה.

Vah-yish-kahv Sh'moo-ayl ahd hah-boh-kehr vah-yeef-tach eht dahl-toht bayt Ah-doh-nai.

And Samuel lay until the morning and opened the doors of the house of the Lord.

—I Samuel 3:15

My soul is woven to my body
With a thread of blood
Flowing through the gateway
Of my heart,
As quietly as the breath
That bends
Through my mouth.

Benefits: This standing pose stretches and strengthens arms, shoulders, lower back, stomach, thighs, and feet. Helps digestion. Calms the mind.

1. Stand up as straight as possible with feet together and arms by your sides. Inhale, and lift your rib cage and chin. Exhale.

2. Inhale, and raise your arms as high as possible. Really stretch your hands toward the ceiling. Look up between your hands.

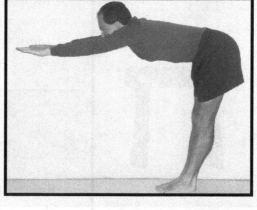

3. Exhale, and slowly reach forward, lowering your arms and back in one straight line until your upper body is parallel to the floor, bending at your hips. Keep looking forward through your hands.

4. Smile, and take three to five deep breaths.

5. Inhaling, slowly raise your upper body, reaching up with your arms.

6. Exhale, and lower your arms.

Hay

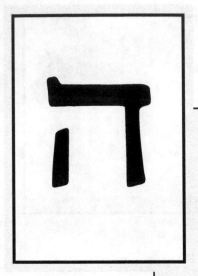

This letter is the symbol for taking. A corresponding yoga pose is *prasarita padottanasana*, the extended foot pose.

בָּרוּךְ אַתָּה יְיָ
הַמַּחֲזִיר נְשָׁמוֹת לִפְגָרִים מֵתִים.

Bah-ruch ah-tah Ah-doh-nai, hah-mah-chah-zeer neh-shah-moht leef-gah-reem may-teem.

Blessed are You, God, who restores souls to dead bodies.

—from the daily prayer book

The body
Without a soul
Lies lifeless,
Nothing to behold.

But with each waking,
Our bodies reunite
With the souls
That animate.

A delicate balance,
Like a hand
Just touching.

Benefits: This standing pose stretches and strengthens feet, ankles, thighs, hips, and lower back. Lengthens the spine and improves posture.

1. Stand up as straight as possible with your arms by your sides. Inhale.

2. Exhale, jump or walk your legs apart 4 feet, and place your hands on your hips. Inhale again.

3. Exhale, and with a straight back, bend at the waist until your upper body is parallel to the floor.

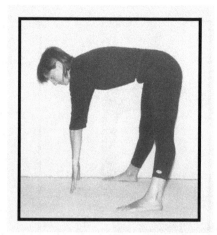

4. Place both hands on the floor, touching with only the fingertips. Keep your head and neck straight, looking down at the floor without bending your neck.

5. Smile, and take three to five deep breaths.

6. Place your hands on your hips. Inhale, and slowly lift your upper body back up straight.

7. Exhale, and jump your feet back together.

Vav

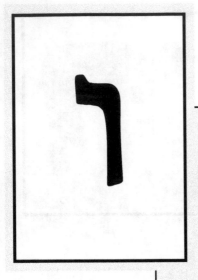

This letter means "and" and symbolizes connection. A corresponding yoga pose is *tadasana,* the mountain pose.

וּבָרָא בוֹ נְקָבִים נְקָבִים
חֲלוּלִים חֲלוּלִים.

Oo-vah-rah voh n'kah-veem n'kah-veem chah-loo-leem chah-loo-leem.

...and has created in us a multitude of openings and organs.

—from the daily prayer book

Our bodies were formed in God's image.
Miraculous machines unequaled in design,
With holes and tubes, nerves and bones,
Muscles and skin, electricity and fluids.
As graceful and perfect as a mountain,
With caves and streams,
And birds and stones.

Benefits: This standing pose stretches and strengthens the feet and knees. Aligns spine for good posture.

1. Stand with your feet together and your arms by your sides.

2. Inhale, and lift your rib cage and chin.

3. Exhale, and relax your shoulders. Your legs should be straight and flexed. Push down through your feet. Imagine a string running through your spine and out the crown of your head. Imagine that someone is pulling the string up so that you grow straighter and taller with each breath.

4. Smile, and take three to five deep breaths.

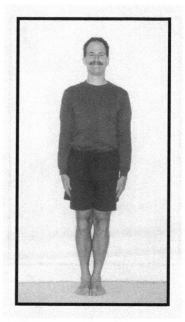

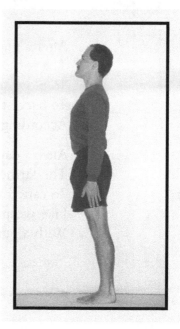

Zayin

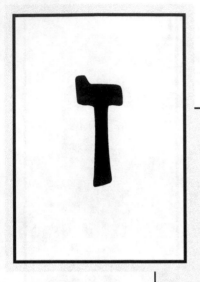

This letter is a symbol for a weapon or "to sustain." A corresponding yoga pose is the rooster, a variation on *tadasana*, the mountain pose.

מַעֲשֶׂיךָ אֲשֶׁר תִּזְרַע בַּשָּׂדֶה.

Mah-ah-seh-chah ah-shehr teez-rah bah-sah-deh.

...the fruits of your work, of what you sow in the field.

—Exodus 23:16

After a night of quiet darkness,
The rooster sets the farmer in motion
To plow and plant,
To harvest and rest,
According to season.

After a day of noise and light,
The farmer renews his strength
To care for his tools,
Like weapons
With a purpose.

Benefits: This standing pose stretches and strengthens the feet and knees. Aligns spine for good posture. Strengthens arms and shoulders.

1. Stand up as straight as possible with your arms by your sides. Inhale.

2. Exhale, and raise your arms so that they are parallel to the floor. Point your fingers down.

3. Inhale, and roll up onto the balls of your feet.

4. Smile, and take three to five deep breaths.

5. Exhale, lower your arms, and come down onto flat feet.

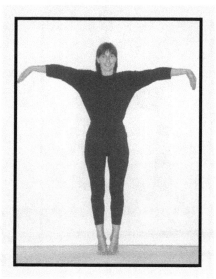

Chet

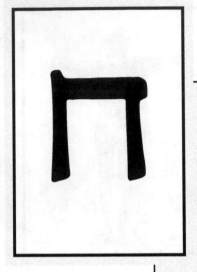

This letter is the symbol for life. A corresponding yoga pose is *ardha chandrasana*, the half moon pose.

וַיִּפַּח בְּאַפָּיו נִשְׁמַת חַיִּים
וַיְהִי הָאָדָם לְנֶפֶשׁ חַיָּה.

Vah-yee-pach b'ah-pahv neesh-maht chah-yeem vah-y'hee hah-ah-dahm l'neh-fesh chah-yah.

God blew into his nostrils the breath of life, and man became a living being.

—Genesis 2:7

I have been given life
For three reasons:
To seek wisdom,
To serve,
And to perform acts
Of lovingkindness.

By the light of the half moon,
I rest
To prepare myself
For another day.

Benefits: This standing pose stretches and strengthens the ankles, legs, hips, lower back, and neck. Lengthens the spine. Develops balance. Improves posture.

1. Stand straight with feet together and arms by your sides. Inhale.

2. Exhale, walk or jump your feet apart 4 feet (as wide as the length of one of your legs), and raise your arms parallel to the floor, palms facing downward.

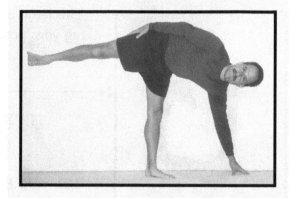

3. Turn your left foot 90 degrees so that the heel of your left foot is in line with the arch of your right foot. Your legs should be straight. Your hips should be facing forward.

4. Inhale, carefully bend your left knee, and reach your left hand down to the floor, placing the fingertips of your left hand 6 to 12 inches ahead of your right foot.

5. Place all your weight on your left leg. Exhale, and then straighten your left leg while lifting your straight right leg completely off the floor. You should be balancing on your left foot and fingertips. Your hips should still be facing forward. Make sure that your right leg is straight and flexed strongly—this will help you balance.

6. Inhale, and place your right arm on your right leg. Look straight ahead or up at the ceiling.

7. Smile, and take three to five deep breaths.

8. Exhale, and slowly lower your straight right leg while bending your left leg.

9. Inhale, and straighten your left leg. Bring your left hand back to your left shin or wherever it comfortably reaches on your left leg. Exhale, and raise your straight right arm back up, pointing toward the ceiling. Both legs should now be straight. You should be back in the triangle pose (see *aleph*).

10. Inhale while reaching up through your right hand. Bring your upper body back to the center with your arms parallel to the floor.

11. Switch feet, and follow steps 1 through 10 on the other side.

12. Inhale, turn both feet so they face forward, and then walk or jump your feet together. Exhale, and lower your arms.

Tet

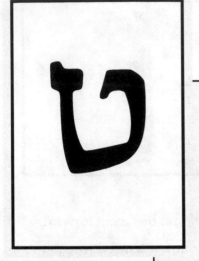

This letter is a symbol for goodness. A corresponding yoga pose is *ardha navasana*, the half boat pose.

וַיַּרְא אֱלֹהִים אֶת כָּל אֲשֶׁר עָשָׂה
וְהִנֵּה טוֹב מְאֹד.

Vah-yahr Eh-loh-heem eht kohl ah-shehr ah-sah v'hee-nay tohv m'ohd.

And God saw all that God had made and found it very good.

—Genesis 1:31

Our bodies formed
In harmony with our surroundings,
With explicit instructions
To tend and to care.

A mission by ship,
To care for the creation.
Land, water, and air,
We hold them all within.

Benefits: This seated pose strengthens the abdomen and lower back. Aids in digestion. Warms the body. Develops balance.

1. Sit on the floor with your legs straight in front of you, your toes pointed forward and your arms at your sides.

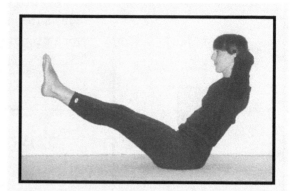

2. Sitting up straight, inhale, bring your hands behind your head, and interlace your fingers.

3. Exhale, and with a straight back, lean your upper body back half way.

4. Simultaneously raise your straight legs together as high as you can. If you have a history of back problems, you should bend your knees before you lift your legs.

5. Smile, and take three to five deep breaths, taking care to keep your back straight and not rounded.

6. Exhale, slowly lower your legs, and sit up straight. Lower your arms.

Yud

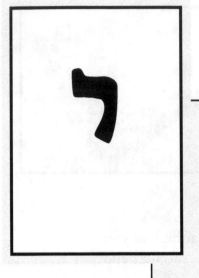

This letter is a symbol for a hand. A corresponding yoga pose is part of the *pawanmuktasana,* the "wind release" exercises for the hands and wrists.

בָּרוּךְ אַתָּה יְיָ אֱלֹהֵינוּ מֶלֶךְ הָעוֹלָם,
אֲשֶׁר קִדְּשָׁנוּ בְּמִצְוֹתָיו
וְצִוָּנוּ עַל נְטִילַת יָדָיִם.

Bah-ruch ah-tah Ah-doh-nai, Eh-loh-hay-noo meh-lech hah-oh-lahm, ah-sher kid-shah-noo b'mitz-voh-tahv v'tzi-vah-noo al ne-ti-laht yah-dah-yim.

Blessed is God, Ruler of the universe, who makes us holy through commandments, and who commands us to raise (wash) our hands.

—from the daily prayer book

By our hands
The world is altered.

Like a farmer's tools,
Our hands work best
When cared for.

Our hands work best
When taking care.

Benefits: These movements stretch and strengthen the wrists, hands, and fingers. Improve circulation and release built-up wastes, or "wind," from joints.

1. Stand up as straight as possible with your arms straight out in front of you.

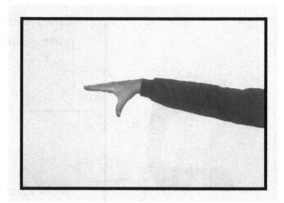

2. Rotate both hands three times to the right and then to the left in wide circles, keeping your elbows straight and locked.

3. With straight arms, extend your hands with palms facing up.

4. Bending only at the wrists, flex your hands and fingers toward you. Inhale. Exhale.

5. Now, open your palms so that they are facing forward, pulling your fingers as far back as possible so that they point to the floor. Inhale. Exhale.

6. Repeat steps 4 and 5 three times.

Kaf

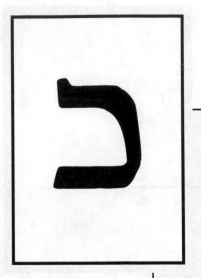

This letter is a symbol for the palm of the hand. A corresponding yoga pose is *janu sirsasana*, the knee-head pose.

כָּל־זְמַן שֶׁהַנְּשָׁמָה בְּקִרְבִּי.

Kohl z'mahn sheh-hah-n'shah-mah b'keer-bee.

...as long as my soul is within me.

—from the daily prayer book

As long as my soul is within me,
I will have the strength
To do what's right.

As long as my soul is within me,
I will care for this body,
For it was a gift.

With palm and knee and head,
Shall I bend to the places
That are hard to reach.

Benefits: This seated pose stretches and strengthens the thighs, knees, lower back, arms, and shoulders. Improves circulation. Calms the mind. Massages the internal organs. Improves digestion.

1. Sit with your legs straight out in front of you. Inhale.

2. Bend your right leg, and place the sole of your right foot on the inside of your left thigh. Exhale, and relax as you let your right knee drop as close to the floor as is comfortable.

3. Inhale, and raise your arms straight up above your head.

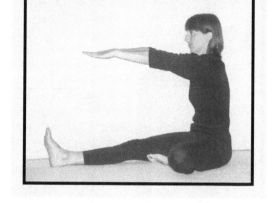

4. Exhale, and lower your arms until they are parallel to the floor.

5. Inhale, and sit up straight. Exhale, and lean forward from your hips. Reach forward as far as you can. To avoid straining your neck, try to touch your chin, rather than your forehead, to your big toe.

6. Smile, and take three to five deep breaths.

7. Inhale, sit up straight, and raise your arms above your head.

8. Exhale, and bring your arms down.

9. Switch legs, and repeat steps 2 through 8.

Final Kaf

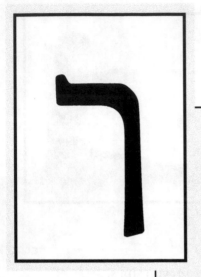

This letter is a symbol for the palm of the hand. A corresponding yoga pose is a variation on *tadasana*, the mountain pose.

וַיֹּאמֶר אֵלָיו יְהוָה לֶךְ־רֵד.

Vah-yoh-mehr ay-lahv Ah-doh-nai lech-rayd.

So the Lord said to him, "Go down (the mountain)."

—Exodus 19:24

To stand still before You,
As a mountain
Stands before the sky,

My body,
Like a mountain
Must be steady,

To balance
The forces acting
In this world.

Benefits: This standing pose stretches and strengthens the knees, ankles, feet, and toes. Strengthens and aligns the spine. Develops good posture. Strengthens the arms and shoulders.

1. Stand with your feet together and your arms by your sides.

2. Inhale, and lift your rib cage and chin.

3. Exhale, and relax your shoulders. Your legs should be straight and flexed. Push down through your feet. Imagine a string running through your spine and out the crown of your head. Imagine that someone is pulling the string up so that you grow straighter and taller with each breath.

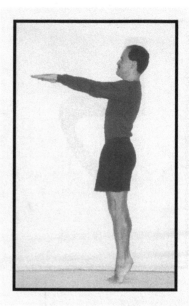

4. Inhale, and raise your arms in front of you until they are parallel to the floor. Look straight ahead.

5. Stand on tiptoes or on the balls of your feet.

6. Smile, and take three to five deep breaths.

7. Exhale, lower your arms, and come down onto flat feet.

Lamed

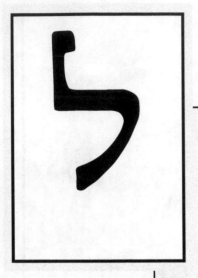

This letter is a symbol of learning or teaching. A corresponding yoga pose is *utkatasana,* the lightning pose.

אִי אֶפְשָׁר לְהִתְקַיֵּם וְלַעֲמוֹד לְפָנֶיךָ.

Ee ehf'shahr l'heet-kah-yaym v'lah-ah-mohd l'fah-neh-chah.

We would be unable to stay alive and stand before You.

—from the daily prayer book

I must learn
To care for this body.
It can teach me
If I learn to listen.

When cared for,
It can strike the earth
Like a shot of lightning,
Electrifying all around.

But if neglected,
I would be unable
To stay alive
And stand before You.

Benefits: This standing pose stretches and strengthens the feet, ankles, knees, thighs, hips, shoulders, and spine.

1. Stand up as straight as possible with your arms by your sides.

2. Inhale, and raise your arms above your head, in line with your torso and with your palms facing each other. Reach as high as you can, stretching your upper back.

3. Without losing the stretch in your upper back, exhale, and bend both legs as much as you can, ideally until your thighs are parallel to the floor. For a deeper stretch, you may lean your torso forward slightly, keeping your back straight. Lean back on your heels, and try to pull your chest up and back.

4. Smile, and take three to five deep breaths.

5. Inhale, and stand up straight.

6. Exhale, and lower your arms.

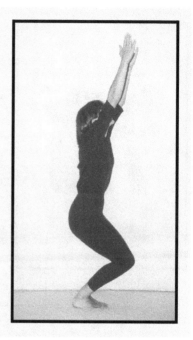

Mem

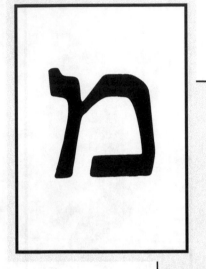

This letter is a symbol for water. A corresponding yoga pose is *ustrasana*, the camel pose.

וַתַּעַן לָהֶם מִרְיָם שִׁירוּ לַיהוָה.

Vah-tah-ahn lah-hem Meer-yahm shee-roo la-Ah-doh-nai.

And Miriam chanted for them: "Sing to God..."

—Exodus 15:21, from the Song of the Sea

Each body is a tent,
A tabernacle,
A dwelling place of Your glory.

Like a camel,
We face each day
Steady, but unsure
When the next oasis will come.

So, like a camel,
Each body must be tended,
To fulfill the master's commandments,
To do good deeds,
To help repair that which is broken.

Benefits: This back-bending pose stretches and strengthens the feet, ankles, shins, knees, thighs, stomach, hips, lower back, chest, neck, arms, and hands. Opens the chest and throat. Energizes the whole body. Expands breathing capacity.

1. Kneel on both knees on the floor with your hips resting on your heels. Inhale.

2. Exhale, and lean backward, placing both palms on the floor with your fingers facing toward your back.

3. Inhale, and lift your hips as high as you can, tightening your buttocks.

4. Look up at the ceiling.

5. Smile, and take three to five deep breaths.

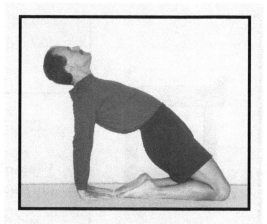

6. On the next exhale, lower your hips back down to your heels.

7. Inhale, and sit up straight.

Final Mem

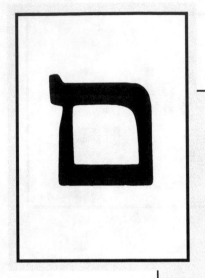

This letter is a symbol for water. A corresponding yoga pose is *paschimottanasana*, the forward bend.

וְרוּחַ אֱלֹהִים מְרַחֶפֶת עַל פְּנֵי הַמָּיִם.

V'roo-ahch Eh-loh-heem m'rah-che-feht ahl p'nay hah-mah-yeem.

...and the spirit of God hovered over the waters.

—Genesis 1:2

A good name reaches forward,
Like a river,
To generations unborn.

A good name reaches backward,
Like a glacier,
To all who brought it to this moment.

The Good Name is here with us all,
Guiding our bodies with choices.

Benefits: This seated pose stretches and strengthens the thighs, knees, lower back, arms, shoulders, and neck. Improves circulation. Calms the mind. Massages internal organs. Improves digestion.

1. Sit with your legs straight out in front of you.

2. Inhale, and raise your arms straight up above your head.

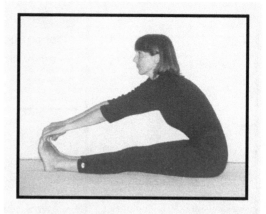

3. Exhale, and reach your arms forward and down until your hands touch some part of your legs or feet.

4. Inhale, and look up to the ceiling. Straighten your back.

5. Exhale, and reach with your chin and hands toward your feet. Try not to round your shoulders.

6. Smile, and take three to five deep breaths, inching forward with your upper body with each exhale.

7. Inhale, and slowly sit up straight.

Nun

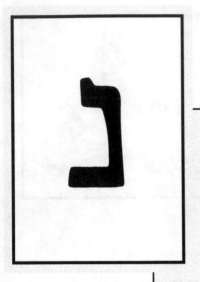

This letter is a symbol of a kingdom or a fish. A corresponding yoga pose is *badha konasana*, the butterfly or cobbler pose.

נְשָׁמָה שֶׁנָּתַתָּ בִּי טְהוֹרָה הִיא.

N'shah-mah sheh-nah-tah-tah bee t'hoh-rah hee.

...the soul You placed within me is pure.

—from the daily prayer book

The human body is an invention
Of unparalleled subtlety and detail,
More delicate than a butterfly,
More streamlined than a fish.

The soul You placed within me is pure,
Animating Your creation
In countless ways.

You breathed life into me
For a purpose in Your kingdom.

Benefits: This seated pose stretches and strengthens the ankles, knees, groin, and hips. Opens the hip joints for leg mobility. Strengthens and aligns the spine.

1. Sit with your legs straight out in front of you. Inhale.

2. Exhale, bend both legs, and place the soles of your feet together.

3. Inhale, interlace your fingers, and clasp them around your toes.

4. Exhale, place your heels as close to your groin as possible, and lower your bent knees as close to the floor as is comfortable.

5. Inhale, lift your rib cage and chin, and sit up as straight as you can.

6. Smile, and take three to five deep breaths.

7. On the last exhale, release your hands and straighten your legs. Shake your legs gently.

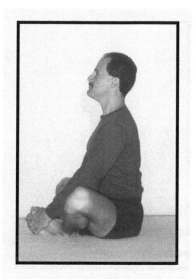

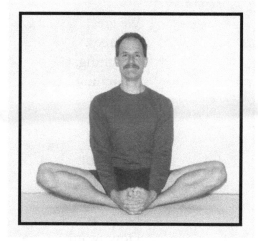

Final Nun

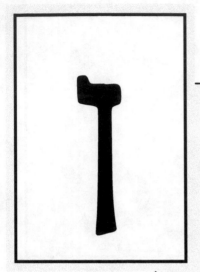

This letter is a symbol for a kingdom or a fish. A corresponding yoga pose is *vrksasana*, the tree pose.

מִבֶּטֶן שְׁאוֹל שִׁוַּעְתִּי שָׁמַעְתָּ קוֹלִי.

Mee-beh-tehn Sh'ohl shee-vah-tee shah-mah-tah koh-lee.

...out of the belly of Sheol I cried, and You heard my voice.

—Jonah 2:3

We are
All trees.
Reaching,
Stretching,
Upward
Toward
Heaven.
Reaching
Up
While
Digging
Downward
Into
The earth.
Marking time
In the circles
We make with our lives.

Benefits: This standing pose stretches the shoulders, feet, and hips. Tones the leg muscles. Aligns the spine. Improves balance and posture.

1. Stand up as straight as possible with your feet together and arms by your sides.

2. Inhale, and place your hands on your hips.

3. While still standing up straight, exhale, and bend your right leg. Reach your right hand down to grasp your right ankle, balancing on your left foot.

4. Inhale, and place the sole of your right foot on your left inner thigh with your toes pointing down. Press your right heel firmly into your left thigh.

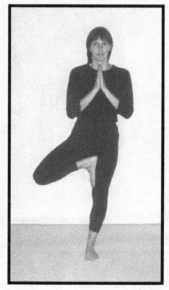

5. Exhale, and let go with your right hand, keeping your right leg bent and your right foot pressing into your left thigh. Bring the palms of your hands together in front of your heart. Keep your back as straight as you can. It will help you to balance if you focus on one spot on the wall.

6. Smile, and take three to five deep breaths.

7. On the last exhale, lower your arms and your right foot.

8. Repeat steps 2 through 7 on the other side.

Samech

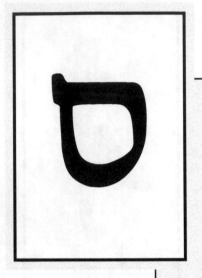

This letter is a symbol of support. A corresponding yoga pose is *dhanurasana*, the bow pose.

אֵין לְשִׁפְחָתְךָ כֹל בַּבַּיִת
כִּי אִם־אָסוּךְ שָׁמֶן.

*Ayn l'sheef-chaht-cha chohl bah-bah-yeet
kee eem ah-sooch shah-mehn.*

**Your servant has nothing in the house,
except a jar of oil.**

—II Kings 4:2

Flesh and bones,
Curved and strong,
Provide a vehicle
For my soul's intent.

Like a bow,
Polished and cared for,
Stays strong and useful
Year after year.

Flesh and bones,
Like a bow,
Support the string
Through which
The archer's energy flows.

Benefits: This lying back-bending pose stretches and strengthens the thighs, lower back, shoulders, neck, and arms. Improves spinal flexibility. Energizes the whole body. Massages the internal organs. Aids digestion.

1. Lie flat on the floor, facing down, with your chin touching the floor and with your palms by your thighs.

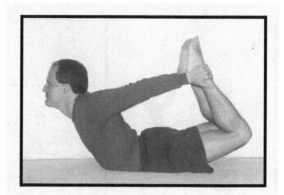

2. Inhale, and bend both legs. Bring your feet as close to your buttocks as possible.

3. Exhale, lift your head, and reach both hands back to grab your feet or ankles.

4. Inhale, and gently raise your feet, legs, head, shoulders, and upper back as high as possible. Try to keep your knees close together.

5. Smile, and take three to five deep breaths.

6. On the last exhale, release your feet and lie flat on the floor with your head turned to the right.

Ayin

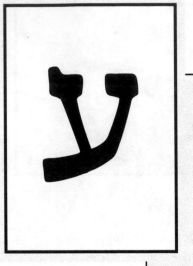

This letter is a symbol for the eye. A corresponding yoga pose is *anantasana,* the leg extension pose.

וְנִפְקְחוּ עֵינֵיכֶם וִהְיִיתֶם כֵּאלֹהִים
יֹדְעֵי טוֹב וָרָע.

V'neef-k'choo ay-nay-chem vee-h'yee-tehm kay-loh-heem yoh-day tohv vah-rah.

...your eyes will be opened and you will be like divine beings who know good and bad.

—Genesis 3:5

In my mind's eye,
I see my legs extended perfectly,
Stretching muscles, tendons, and skin.

How effortlessly
I move my legs
when I walk or sit or lie.

Only in times of discomfort
Do I seem to notice
Their presence.

Rarely
Do I sense the wonder
Of their extraordinary design.

Benefits: This lying pose stretches and strengthens the legs, hips, waist, and neck. Improves circulation.

1. Lie on your left side with your head propped up on your left elbow and hand.

2. Inhale, and raise your straight right leg as high as you can.

3. Exhale, and raise your right arm up straight toward the ceiling. If you are flexible, try grabbing your right big toe with your right index finger and then straightening your leg.

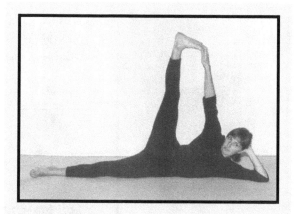

4. Smile, and take three to five deep breaths.

5. On your last exhale, release your toe and lower your leg.

6. Roll onto your right side, and repeat steps 1 through 5.

Pey

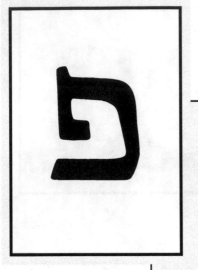

This letter is a symbol for a mouth. A corresponding yoga pose is a beginning position for *kapotasana*, the pigeon pose.

לֹא תוּכַל לִרְאֹת אֶת־פָּנָי
כִּי לֹא־יִרְאַנִי הָאָדָם וָחָי.

Loh too-chahl leer-oht eht pah-nai kee loh yeer-ah-nee hah-ah-dahm vah-chai.

...you cannot see My face, for man may not see My face and live.

—Exodus 33:20

Bodies bend and flex,
Curved
Like a mouth
Alternately
Smiling
And frowning.

When I close my eyes,
I look inward.
I sit up straight,
Face to face with God.
Eyes closed,
Therefore, I live.

Benefits: This back-bending pose stretches and strengthens the neck, lower back, abdomen, hips, legs, feet, and ankles. Opens the throat and chest. Deepens breathing.

1. Kneel on the floor with your thighs perpendicular to the floor.

2. Inhale, and raise your right arm. Exhale, reach back, and rest your right hand on your right hip with your fingers pointing up or away from the body.

3. Inhale, and raise the left arm up. Exhale, reach back, and rest your left hand on your left hip with your fingers pointing up or away from the body.

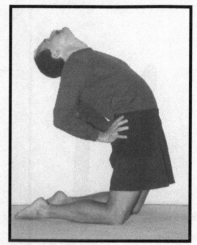

4. Inhale, and cover your top lip with your bottom lip so that you do not strain your neck. Exhale, and gently lean your head, neck, and shoulders back until you are looking at the ceiling. Your hands should press your pelvis forward gently.

5. Smile, and take three to five deep breaths.

6. Inhale, and come back up to kneeling.

7. Exhale, and lower your hands to your sides.

Final Pey

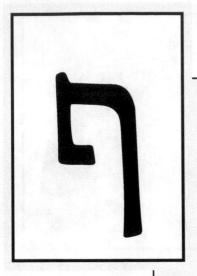

This letter is a symbol of a mouth. A corresponding yoga pose is an intermediate position of *urdhva dhanurasana*, the standing back-bend.

עֲבַדְתִּיךָ אַרְבַּע־עֶשְׂרֵה שָׁנָה
בִּשְׁתֵּי בְנֹתֶךָ וְשֵׁשׁ שָׁנִים בְּצֹאנֶךָ
וַתַּחֲלֵף אֶת־מַשְׂכֻּרְתִּי עֲשֶׂרֶת מֹנִים.

Ah-vahd-tee-chah ahr-bah ehs-ray shah-nah beesh-tay v'noh-teh-chah v'shaysh shah-neem b'tzoh-neh-chah vah-tah-chah-layf eht mahs-koor-tee ah-seh-reht moh-neem.

"I served you fourteen years for your two daughters, and six years for your flocks, and you changed my wages time and again."

—Genesis 31:41

Bending forward,
Bending backward,
Reaching from side to side.
We move our bodies
To change the world
Without end.

Lying, sitting, speaking, standing, walking—work.
Sitting, speaking, standing, walking—home.
Sitting, speaking, standing,
Sitting, speaking, lying down,
We move our bodies and our mouths
To serve You
Without end.

Benefits: This standing back-bend stretches and strengthens the front of the torso. Opens the throat and chest. Expands lung capacity. Strengthens the lower back and legs.

1. Stand up as straight as possible with your arms by your sides.

2. Inhale, and raise your right arm straight up. Exhale, and reach back, placing your right hand on your right hip with your fingers pointing up or away from the side of your body.

3. Inhale, and raise your left arm straight up. Exhale, and reach back, placing your left hand on your left hip with your fingers pointing up or away from the side of your body.

4. Cover your top lip with your bottom lip to protect your neck, and then gently lean your head, neck, and shoulders back until you are looking at the ceiling. Your hands should press your pelvis forward gently.

5. Smile, and take three to five deep breaths.

6. Inhale, and slowly stand up straight.

7. Exhale, and release your hands.

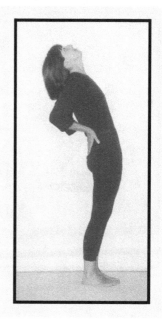

Tzadi

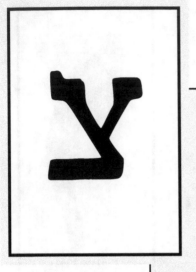

This letter is a symbol of righteousness or the hunt. A corresponding yoga pose is *urdhva prasarita padasana*, the upright extended foot pose.

וַיֹּאמֶר אֱלֹהִים נַעֲשֶׂה אָדָם בְּצַלְמֵנוּ כִּדְמוּתֵנוּ.

Vah-yoh-mehr Eh-loh-heem nah-ah-seh ah-dahm b'tzahl-may-noo keed-moo-tay-noo.

And God said, "Let us make man in our image, after our likeness."

—Genesis 1:26

Moses was human,
A seeker, a righteous man.
With the strength of his hand,
He held the staff
That split the rock
And the sea.

With the strength of his legs,
He stood on holy ground.
He wandered deserts
And climbed Mount Sinai,
Time and time again.

And with the strength of his spirit,
He yearned for Zion.

Benefits: This inverted pose strengthens the abdomen, hips, and legs. Reduces fat around the waist. Warms the body. Massages the internal organs. Improves circulation.

1. Lie flat on your back with your hands palms down on the floor.

2. Inhale, and raise your legs together until they are perpendicular to the floor.

3. Exhale, and slowly lower your right leg halfway down, keeping your left leg straight up.

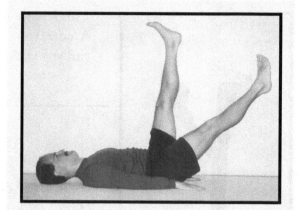

4. Smile, and take three to five deep breaths.

5. Inhale, and raise your right leg back to straight up.

6. Repeat steps 3, 4, and 5 with your left leg.

7. Exhale, and slowly lower both legs to the floor.

Final Tzadi

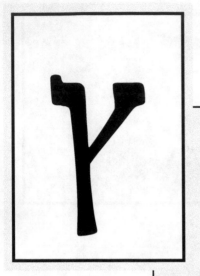

This letter is a symbol of righteousness or the hunt. A corresponding yoga pose is *utthita hasta padangusthasana*, the extended hand and foot pose.

עֵץ־חַיִּים הִיא לַמַּחֲזִיקִים בָּהּ.

Aytz chah-yeem hee lah-mah-cha-zee-keem bah.

She (wisdom) is a tree of life to those who lay hold upon her.

—Proverbs 3:18

The tree of life
Has many branches.
All reaching
With arms and hands and fingers.

The tree of life
Has many roots.
All holding
The same ground.

Benefits: This standing pose stretches and strengthens the legs, hips, arms, and shoulders. Tones the thighs. Opens the hip joints for leg mobility.

1. Stand up as straight as possible with your arms by your sides and with your left hip next to the back of a chair, sturdy shelf, or window ledge that is higher than your hip. Take one step to the right so that you are approximately 3 feet from the chair, shelf, or ledge.

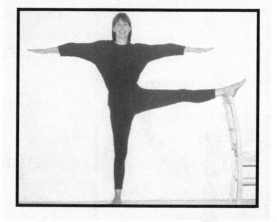

2. Inhale, and place your hands on your hips.

3. Exhale, lift your left leg sideways to the left, and carefully place your left heel on the back of the chair, ledge, or shelf.

4. Inhale, and raise your arms out to your sides until they are parallel to the floor. Reach out through your fingertips. Straighten your spine, lifting up through your head. Keep your right leg straight. Look forward.

5. Smile, and take three to five deep breaths.

6. On your last exhale, lower your arms and your leg from the chair.

7. Repeat steps 1 through 6 on the right side.

Kuf

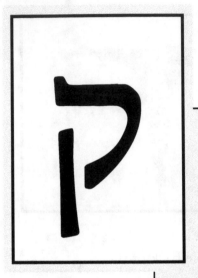

This letter is a symbol for a monkey or "to surround." A corresponding yoga pose is *pranatasana*, the child's pose.

וַתִּקַּח נָעֳמִי אֶת־הַיֶּלֶד
וַתְּשִׁתֵהוּ בְחֵיקָהּ וַתְּהִי־לוֹ לְאֹמֶנֶת.

Vah-tee-kach Nah-ah-mee eht hah-yeh-lehd vat-shee-tay-hoo v'chay-kah vaht-hee loh l'oh-meh-neht.

Then Naomi took the child and laid him in her bosom.

—Ruth 4:16

With intention, we move our bodies forward
In a direction of health.
We have been crowned with a thinking brain.

Yet, the monkey does not over-eat
Or sit too long in front of a lighted screen.
The rabbit does not forget
To stretch its legs.

Your lovingkindness is forever.
It surrounds us and is strengthened
When we strengthen ourselves.

Benefits: This lying pose stretches the lower back, shoulders, arms, shins, and ankles. Massages the internal organs. Calms the mind.

1. Kneel on both knees on the floor with your buttocks touching your heels and your feet pointing backward, soles facing upward. Inhale.

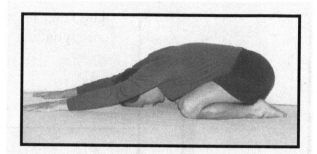

2. Exhale, and lean your upper body forward until your forehead touches the floor.

3. Inhale, and reach your arms forward, palms facing down on the floor.

4. Relax, and take three to five deep breaths.

5. Inhale, and sit back up on your heels.

Raysh

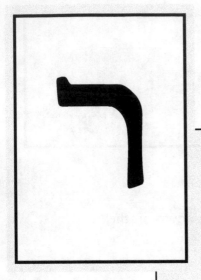

This letter is a symbol of a head or a beginning. A corresponding yoga pose is *nitambhasana*, the reed.

רוֹפֵא כָל בָּשָׂר.

Ro-fay chohl bah-sahr.

...who heals all flesh.

—from the daily prayer book

In our beginning,
You breathed life into our form.
At the impact of our parents' bodies,
You were there with us.
You, who heals all flesh,
Help us learn to heal ourselves.
Help us to bend,
Rather than break,
Like a reed.

Benefits: This standing pose stretches the rib cage, lower back, and waist. Trims fat from the sides. Opens the rib cage. Deepens breathing.

1. Stand up as straight as possible with your arms by your sides.

2. Inhale, and raise your arms, reaching as high as you can. Try to bring your palms together, but keep your arms straight. If this is too much of a stretch, keep your arms shoulder width apart.

3. Exhale, and lean your upper body to the right as far as you can, keeping your arms straight and your biceps touching your ears. Keep your feet planted firmly on the floor.

4. Smile, and take three to five deep breaths, stretching your side a little more with each exhale.

5. Inhale, stand up straight, and lower your arms.

6. Repeat steps 2 through 5 on the left side.

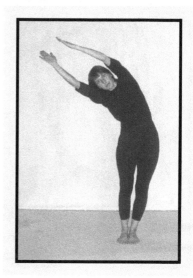

Shin

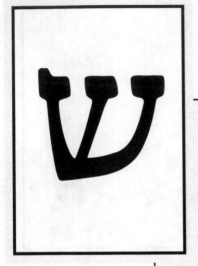

This letter is a symbol for a tooth or change. A corresponding yoga pose is *salabhasana I,* the inverted boat.

שֶׁהֶחֱזַרְתָּ בִּי נִשְׁמָתִי בְּחֶמְלָה.

Sheh-heh-cheh-zahr-tah bee neesh-mah-tee b'chehm-lah.

You have restored my soul to me with mercy.

—from the daily prayer book

Each night I lie in my ark,
Floating among the reeds of dreams.
Hoping to wake the next morning
With the strength to make a change.

Each morning I give thanks
That You have restored my soul to me.
With mercy You have reunited
Flesh and spirit
In peace.

Benefits: This lying pose stretches and strengthens the neck, shoulders, arms, hips, lower back, legs, and feet. Energizes the whole body. Massages the internal organs. Aids digestion.

1. Lie flat on the floor, face down, with your feet together, your chin on the floor, and your palms face down by your hips.

2. Reach your hands behind your back, and clasp your hands.

3. Inhale, and raise your upper body and head off the floor by pulling back with your hands. Simultaneously bend your legs, lifting and pointing your feet toward the ceiling.

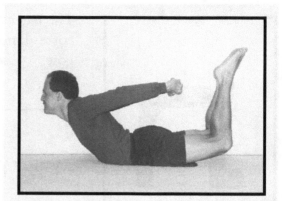

4. Smile, and take three to five deep breaths.

5. On the last exhale, lower your legs and then your upper body.

6. Turn your head to the left and release your arms, placing them palms down by your sides. Rest for a few breaths.

7. To come out of the pose, roll onto your right side, and sit up.

Tav

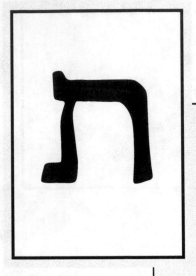

This letter is a symbol for a sign or an impression. A corresponding yoga pose is *marjarasana*, the cat pose.

אֶת־קַשְׁתִּי נָתַתִּי בֶּעָנָן
וְהָיְתָה לְאוֹת בְּרִית בֵּינִי וּבֵין הָאָרֶץ.

Eht kahsh-tee nah-tah-tee beh-ah-nahn v'hai-tah l'oht b'reet bay-nee oo-vayn hah-ah-rehtz.

"I have set My bow in the clouds, and it will serve as a sign of the covenant between Me and the earth."

—Genesis 9:13

Each morning is an answer,
A return to the world in need
Of my efforts.

Each morning is a sign
That our efforts are needed.

I stretch like a cat,
And then I am ready
To make a difference.

Benefits: This lying/back-bending pose stretches and strengthens the abdomen, spine, and neck. Provides a gentle massage to the internal organs. Aids digestion.

1. Lie flat on the floor, face down.

2. Inhale, and place your hands under your shoulders, palms down.

3. Exhale, and push yourself up onto your hands and knees. Your arms should be straight and perpendicular to the floor.

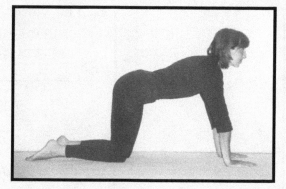

4. Inhale, and look up at the ceiling, curving your back toward the floor, lengthening your stomach, and drawing your hips back toward your feet.

5. Exhale while tucking your chin to your chest and arching your back toward the ceiling, pushing the air out of your lungs by contracting your stomach and diaphragm strongly. Pull your hips forward toward your arms.

6. Repeat steps 4 and 5 four more times. To stretch different areas of the back, you can vary the distance between your hands and your knees.

Kamatz

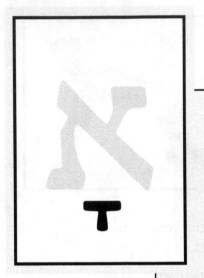

This vowel has the sound "ah." A corresponding yoga pose is *jathara parivartanasana*, the stomach-turning pose.

וּמַעֲשֵׂהֶם כַּאֲשֶׁר יִהְיֶה הָאוֹפָן בְּתוֹךְ הָאוֹפָן.

Oo-mah-ah-say-hehm kah-ah-shehr yee-h'yeh hah-oh-fahn b'tohch hah-oh-fahn.

...and their work was as it were a wheel within a wheel.

—Ezekiel 1:16

Time and space are curved.
Moments twist and turn,
Making their way
Through the tunnels
Formed at the instant of creation.

In the subatomic world within us,
Matter turns to energy
And back again,
As fast as the speed of light
Squared.

On the eternal wheel,
All are created and destroyed,
Only to be reborn
On the next turn.

Benefits: This twisting pose gently realigns the spine after the bending movements of the other poses. As it twists the abdomen it massages the internal organs, helping squeeze waste products from the tissues and improve digestion.

1. Lie flat on your back with your arms extended like a "T" and your feet together.

2. Inhale, and raise your knees together toward your chest.

3. As you exhale, slowly lower your knees to the right side—all the way to the floor if you can—but don't force. Keep your shoulders on the floor.

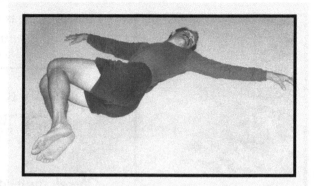

4. Take a deep breath, and slowly turn your head to the left. Take three to five deep breaths.

5. Inhale, and bring your head and knees to the center.

6. Repeat steps 3 through 5 on the other side.

Patach

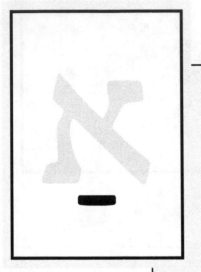

This vowel has the sound "ah." A corresponding yoga pose is *savasana*, the corpse pose.

עֹשֶׂה שָׁלוֹם בִּמְרוֹמָיו הוּא יַעֲשֶׂה
שָׁלוֹם עָלֵינוּ וְעַל־כָּל־יִשְׂרָאֵל
וְאִמְרוּ אָמֵן.

*Oh-seh shah-lohm beem-roh-mahv hoo
yah-ah-seh shah-lohm ah-lay-noo v'ahl
kohl yees-rah-ayl v'eem-roo ah-mayn.*

May God who causes peace to reign in the
high heavens, let peace descend on us, on all
Israel, and all the world, and let us say: Amen.

—from the daily prayer book

Lying like a corpse,
A body here and now.
Breathing noiselessly,
Releasing the hold
Of muscle on bone.

Lying flat
Face up to the sky,
Back down to the earth,
Quietly connected
To everything.

Benefits: This simple lying pose helps reduce
fatigue and quiet the mind. It expands awareness of
the body and breath, particularly when it follows the
work of the other poses. It helps to integrate the
effects of the other poses by allowing the muscles
and tendons to relax completely and the breathing
to normalize without movement of the body.

This pose should be done at the end of every yoga session. Relax in savasana *for 5 minutes for every half-hour of practicing poses.*

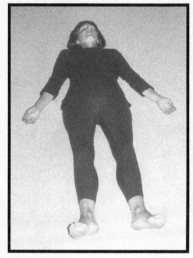

1. Lie on your back with your legs about 6 inches apart, hands by your sides, palms facing upward. Close your eyes. Let your body relax onto the floor.

2. Consciously slow your breathing. Try to breathe so quietly that someone next to you could not hear you breathing.

3. Mentally scan your body from your feet to your face, relaxing each part of your body as you think of it. Relax your ankles. Relax your knees and thighs. Relax your hips and lower back. Relax your upper back, shoulders, arms, elbows, and hands. Relax your neck. Relax your scalp, face, eyes, and jaw. Breathe quietly, and let yourself relax. Try not to fall asleep. Be aware of yourself.

4. With your eyes closed, try to look at the inside of your forehead. Try to quiet your mind and clear it of all thoughts. Or focus on your breathing, on the way your breath rises and falls in your belly. Feel your connection to the floor growing as you relax deeper and deeper. Feel your connection to the air you are breathing.

5. When you are ready, come out of this relaxation pose slowly. With your eyes still closed, wiggle your toes and fingers. Roll your head gently from side to side. Roll onto your right side, and bend your knees so that you are in the fetal position. Take a few deep breaths. Slowly sit up to a cross-legged position. Open your eyes. Try to remember that peaceful feeling for the rest of the day. Shalom.

4 ◈ The Aleph-Bet Yoga Series— the Proper Order of a Yoga Session

Yoga poses are generally done as a series of complementary and counter-balancing movements. Although each yoga posture can be practiced individually, when you practice several poses at one time, you should follow a set order. In this chapter, the yoga poses are presented in the order of a balanced yoga practice session: what I call the Aleph-Bet Yoga series, rather than simply arranged in the order of the Hebrew *aleph-bet* as shown in chapter 3.

Yoga poses are usually grouped into categories, such as standing, sitting, or lying. In most styles of hatha yoga, the pose categories are taught in a particular order, with a variety of poses from each category practiced in each session. Several poses of one category are usually practiced together before the person moves on to another category. To provide the maximum benefits and prevent injury, poses are balanced or completed by poses that stretch in the opposite direction. For example, poses that bend the body forward are paired with poses that bend the body backward; poses that strengthen the abdomen are paired with poses that strengthen the back; poses that stretch one side are followed by the same pose on the opposite side.

A typical series of hatha yoga poses begins by working the arms and legs through the standing and sitting poses. These poses stretch and strengthen the joints and their supporting muscles and tendons. They also help increase blood circulation from the outer extremities to the heart. For the same reason, some styles of yoga begin a session with more completely inverted poses, like the headstand and shoulder stand (which are not shown in this book). After the standing, sitting, and inverted poses, it is common to work the middle of the body with lying poses, back-bends, and twists. These types of poses stretch and massage the internal organs, including the spinal cord and major nerve branches, and stretch and strengthen the muscles and tissues that protect those organs. These types of poses are often alternated as counter-stretches to each other to prevent strain to one side of the body or the other. For example, *marjarasana*, the cat pose, is often used to counter-stretch kneeling back-bends like *ustrasana*, the camel pose.

Back-bending poses energize the whole body. They release stored tension in the back and neck, stimulating the brain and body and increasing one's feeling of overall well-being. In this way, back-bending poses are also helpful in treating depression. Twisting poses also help realign the spine after the intense stretching movements of the other poses.

Finally, every hatha yoga session should end with a deep relaxation, such as *savasana*, the corpse pose. It is very important to follow the movements of the poses with a relaxation pose that lasts at least 5 minutes for every half-hour of practicing poses. A relaxation pose can be done at any time and helps reduce fatigue and quiet the mind. Deep relaxation expands awareness of the body, particularly when it follows the work of the other poses. It helps integrate the effects of the other poses by allowing the muscles and tendons to recover and the breathing to normalize before one goes back to other activities.

In this chapter, I have organized the yoga poses and corresponding Hebrew letters into a series of poses called the Aleph-Bet Yoga series. The Aleph-Bet Yoga series is appropriate for beginners but also challenging for people who are familiar with the basic hatha yoga postures. The Aleph-Bet Yoga series begins with standing poses, then moves to sitting poses and an inverted pose, followed by a combination of back-bends, lying poses, and twists. Use the descriptions of how to do each of the poses from chapter 3, but follow the order presented here in chapter 4. Once you learn the basic techniques of the poses described in chapter 3, the series should take you approximately 30 to 45 minutes.

If you are experienced with hatha yoga then I recommend that you do all the poses each time, adding other poses that you know for additional benefit. If you are just beginning, or if you do not have time to do the whole series, you may choose to focus on just a few letter poses in each session, or you may skip some poses that are similar within one of the categories. While you are learning the basics, or just for variety, you may want to vary the poses in a particular grouping each day. It is all right to shorten the session, but please do not skip the concluding relaxation pose. If you would like a shorter session, I recommend following the guidelines at the end of this chapter regarding substitutions.

Before you get started with the series, here's one final note about breathing. In hatha yoga, breathing correctly is as important as practicing the correct form of the posture. We draw our energy from food and from the air we breathe, and learning how to breathe correctly can help us to make the most of the potential energy we can obtain from these sources. Entire books have been written on the various breathing techniques, known in hatha yoga as *pranayama,* ranging from simple to complex. I will not discuss anything complicated here; for that you should find an experienced teacher. But I would like to suggest a very simple breathing exercise as a warm-up before you begin any series of postures.

First, stand up straight but relaxed, with your arms by your sides. Your knees can be bent slightly. Turn your palms to face forward, and begin inhaling through your nose as you reach your arms up toward the ceiling, bringing your palms together or facing each other from shoulder width. Inhale as much as you can—fill your lungs completely. When you finish the inhale, turn your palms away from each other and begin exhaling while lowering your arms back to your sides. Exhale as completely as you can. On the next inhale, as you raise your arms, look up to the ceiling. As you exhale, lower your gaze toward the floor as you lower your arms. Repeat these movements with complete breathing three times. You may try bending and straightening your knees in coordination with your arm movements: straightening as you inhale and bring your arms up, bending as you exhale and bring your arms down. As you move into practicing the series of postures, try to keep this breathing rhythm. Keep your breaths long and complete. Inhale fully. Exhale fully.

Name and Page Number of the Hatha Yoga Pose	Figure of the Yoga Pose	Category of Pose	Hebrew Character
1. *Tadasana*, the mountain pose—see page 33 for technique		Standing	ו
2. *Tadasana* variation, the rooster pose—see page 35 for technique		Standing	ז
3. *Nitambhasana*, the reed pose—see page 71 for technique		Standing	ר
4. *Uttanasana* variation, the forward extension pose—see page 29 for technique		Standing	ד
5. *Urdhva dhanurasana* variation, the standing back-bend with hands on buttocks—see page 63 for technique		Standing	ק
6. *Tadasana* variation, the mountain pose variation with arms extended—see page 45 for technique		Standing	ך

Name and Page Number of the Hatha Yoga Pose	Figure of the Yoga Pose	Category of Pose	Hebrew Character
7. *Pawanmuktasana,* the wind-releasing series for the hands and wrists—see page 41 for technique		Standing	ר
8. *Vrksasana,* the tree pose—see page 55 for technique		Standing	ז
9. *Utkatasana,* the lightning pose—see page 47 for technique		Standing	ל
10. *Virabhadrasana* variation, the warrior I pose—see page 27 for technique		Standing	ג
11. *Utthita trikonasana,* the triangle pose—see page 23 for technique		Standing	א
12. *Ardha chandrasana,* the half moon pose—see page 37 for technique		Standing	ח

Name and Page Number of the Hatha Yoga Pose	Figure of the Yoga Pose	Category of Pose	Hebrew Character
13. *Prasarita padottanasana* variation, the extended foot pose— see page 31 for technique		Standing	ה
14. *Utthita hasta padangusthasana*, the extended hand and foot pose— see page 67 for technique		Standing	צ
15. *Dandasana* variation, the stick pose with arms extended—see page 25 for technique		Sitting	ב
16. *Janu sirsasana* variation, knee-head pose—see page 43 for technique		Sitting	כ
17. *Paschimottanasana*, the forward bend—see page 51 for technique		Sitting	ם
18. *Badha konasana*, the cobbler or butterfly pose—see page 53 for technique		Sitting	נ
19. *Ardha navasana*, the half boat pose—see page 39 for technique		Sitting	ט

Name and Page Number of the Hatha Yoga Pose	Figure of the Yoga Pose	Category of Pose	Hebrew Character
20. *Urdhva prasarita padasana* variation, the upright extended foot pose—see 65 for technique		Inverted	
21. *Anantasana,* the leg extension pose—see page 59 for technique	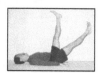	Lying	
22. *Kapotasana* variation, the start of the pigeon pose with hands on buttocks—see page 61 for technique		Back-bending	
23. *Ustrasana* variation, the camel pose—see page 49 for technique		Back-bending	
24. *Marjarasana,* the cat pose—see page 75 for technique	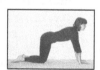	Lying	
25. *Salabhasana I,* the inverted boat pose—see page 73 for technique	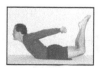	Lying	
26. *Dhanurasana,* the bow pose—see page 57 for technique	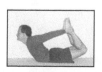	Lying	

Name and Page Number of the Hatha Yoga Pose	Figure of the Yoga Pose	Category of Pose	Hebrew Character
27. *Pranatasana*, the child's pose— see page 69 for technique	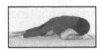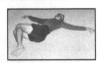	Lying	
28. *Jathara parivartanasana*, stomach-turning pose— see page 77 for technique		Twisting	
29. *Savasana*, the corpse pose— see page 79 for technique		Lying	

Guidelines for Substitutions or Changes to the Aleph-Bet Yoga Series

For a shorter session, I suggest the following alternatives to the full series. Choose one or more of the three standing poses that are based on *tadasana*, the mountain pose (*vav, zayin,* or final *kaf*), instead of doing all three in one session. Do all the poses for *raysh, dalet,* final *pey, yud,* final *nun, lamed,* and *gimmel.* Choose either *aleph* or *chet.* Choose either *hay* or final *tzadi.* Choose one or more of the three sitting forward-bending poses (final *mem, bet,* or *kaf*). Do the poses for *nun* and *tet.* Choose either *pey* or *mem.* Do the pose for *tav.* Choose either the pose for *shin* or the pose for *samech.* And finish with the pose for *kuf,* followed by the poses for *kamatz* and *patach.* This alternative session should take you approximately 20 minutes.

The information I have included in this book is only a basic introduction to yoga and the Hebrew letters. If you wish to learn more about these subjects, I recommend exploring the following resources:

Books

On Judaism

Boorstein, Sylvia. *That's Funny, You Don't Look Buddhist*. San Francisco: HarperCollins, 1997.

Cooper, David A. *Renewing Your Soul: A Guided Retreat for the Sabbath and Other Days of Rest*. San Francisco: Harper San Francisco, 1995. (Revised and reissued as *The Handbook of Jewish Meditation Practices: A Guide for Enriching the Sabbath and Other Days of Your Life*. Woodstock, Vt.: Jewish Lights, 2000.)

————. *Three Gates to Meditation Practice: A Personal Journey into Sufism, Buddhism, and Judaism*. Woodstock, Vt.: SkyLight Paths, 2000.

Davis, Avram, ed. *Meditation from the Heart of Judaism: Today's Teachers Share Their Practices, Techniques, and Faith*. Woodstock, Vt.: Jewish Lights, 1999.

————. *The Way of Flame: A Guide to the Forgotten Mystical Tradition of Jewish Meditation*. Woodstock, Vt.: Jewish Lights, 1999.

Frankiel, Tamar, and Judy Greenfeld. *Entering the Temple of Dreams: Jewish Prayers, Movements, and Meditations for the End of the Day*. Woodstock, Vt.: Jewish Lights, 2000.

————. *Minding the Temple of the Soul: Balancing Body, Mind, and Spirit through Traditional Jewish Prayer, Movement, and Meditation.* Woodstock, Vt.: Jewish Lights, 1997.

Gefen, Nan Fink. *Discovering Jewish Meditation: Instruction & Guidance for Learning an Ancient Spiritual Practice.* Woodstock, Vt.: Jewish Lights, 2000.

Kushner, Lawrence. *The Book of Letters: A Mystical Hebrew Alphabet,* 2nd ed. Woodstock, Vt.: Jewish Lights, 1990.

————. *Honey from the Rock: An Introduction to Jewish Mysticism.* Special Anniversary Edition. Woodstock, Vt.: Jewish Lights, 2000.

Matlins, Stuart M., ed. *The Jewish Lights Spirituality Handbook: A Guide to Understanding, Exploring & Living a Spiritual Life.* Woodstock, Vt.: Jewish Lights, 2001.

On Yoga

Iyengar, B. K. S. *Light on Yoga.* New York: Schocken Books, 1979.

————. *Yoga: The Path to Holistic Health,* London: Dorling Kindersley, 2001.

Lidell, Lucy, and Narayani and Giris Rabinovitch. *The Sivananda Companion to Yoga: A Complete Guide to the Physical Postures, Breathing Exercises, Diet, Relaxation and Meditation Techniques of Yoga.* New York: Simon and Schuster, 1983.

Mehta, Silva, Mira, and Shyam. *Yoga the Iyengar Way: The New Definitive Illustrated Guide.* New York: Alfred A. Knopf, 1990.

Van Lysebeth, Andre. *Yoga Self-Taught.* York Beach, Maine: Samuel Weiser, 1999.

Videotapes

Watching a videotape can be a very useful supplement to yoga classes and books. There are many great yoga videos on the market today. Here are just a few of my favorites. They can be purchased at retail stores or ordered by phone or Internet from Amazon.com or at the numbers or web addresses listed below.

Aerobic Yoga: The Flow Series, with Ganga White and Tracey Rich, by White Lotus Foundation—(805) 964-1944.

Total Yoga, with Ganga White and Tracey Rich, by White Lotus Foundation.

Yoga Journal's series of videotapes by Healing Arts, including:

> *Yoga Journal's Practice Introduction*
> *Yoga Journal's Practice for Beginners*
> *Yoga Journal's Practice for Intermediates*
> *Yoga Journal's Practice for Flexibility*
> *Yoga Journal's Practice for Strength*
> *Yoga Journal's Practice for Relaxation*
> *Yoga Journal's Practice for Energy*
> *Yoga Journal's Practice for Meditation*

YogaKids, with Marsha Wenig, by Living Arts—1 (800) 2-LIVING.

Magazines

These two magazines are extremely useful for getting the perspective of the many styles and teachers of the different kinds of yoga. They contain insightful articles on a range of topics, from natural healing, to events and workshops, to descriptions of individual poses and how to approach them at various levels of ability.

Yoga International—Published bimonthly. For subscription information, contact *Yoga International* at RR1, Box 1130, Honesdale, PA 18431-9718. Or phone them at (570) 253-6243. Fax: (570) 253-6360. E-mail: subscriptions@yimag.org.

Yoga Journal—Published bimonthly with one special additional winter issue. For subscription information, call 1-800-600-YOGA or go to the *Yoga Journal* website at: http://www.yogajournal.com.

Websites

http://www.angelfire.com/pe/ophanim—This website contains information about the *Ophanim,* the name for a specific system of "sacred" physical postures and internal exercises based on the Hebrew alphabet and Jewish mystical tradition.

http://www.dnai.com/~goldfarb/otiyot/—This website contains information about the *Otiyot Khayyot,* or Living Letters, which is a series of gentle, flowing movements based on the shape of the Hebrew letters created by tai chi master and spiritual philosopher Yehudit Goldfarb.

http://www.yogasite.com/index.html—Great general yoga site with connections to lots of useful information and links, including teacher directories, yoga products, and books.

NOTES

NOTES

1. Rabbi Lawrence Kushner, *Honey from the Rock: An Introduction to Jewish Mysticism*, Special Anniversary Edition (Woodstock, Vt.: Jewish Lights, 2000), p. 43.

2. B. K. S. Iyengar, *Light on Yoga* (New York: Schocken Books, 1979), p. 21.

3. Ibid.

4. Ibid.

5. Kushner, *The Book of Letters: A Mystical Hebrew Alphabet,* 2nd ed. (Woodstock, Vt.: Jewish Lights, 1990), p. 17.

6. David A. Cooper, *Renewing Your Soul: A Guided Retreat for the Sabbath and Other Days of Rest* (San Francisco: Harper San Francisco, 1995), pp. 90–117.

7. Iyengar, *Light on Yoga*, p. 22.

Bible Study/Midrash

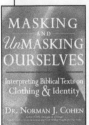

The Book of Job: Annotated & Explained
Translation and Annotation by Donald Kraus; Foreword by Dr. Marc Brettler
Clarifies for today's readers what Job is, how to overcome difficulties in the text, and what it may mean for us. Features fresh translation and probing commentary.
5½ x 8½, 220 pp (est), Quality PB, 978-1-59473-389-5 **$16.99**

Masking and Unmasking Ourselves: Interpreting Biblical Texts on Clothing & Identity *By Dr. Norman J. Cohen*
Presents ten Bible stories that involve clothing in an essential way, as a means of learning about the text, its characters and their interactions.
6 x 9, 240 pp, HC, 978-1-58023-461-0 **$24.99**

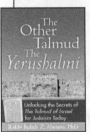

The Other Talmud—*The Yerushalmi*: Unlocking the Secrets of The Talmud of Israel for Judaism Today *By Rabbi Judith Z. Abrams, PhD*
A fascinating—and stimulating—look at "the other Talmud" and the possibilities for Jewish life reflected there. 6 x 9, 256 pp, HC, 978-1-58023-463-4 **$24.99**

The Torah Revolution: Fourteen Truths That Changed the World
By Rabbi Reuven Hammer, PhD A unique look at the Torah and the revolutionary teachings of Moses embedded within it that gave birth to Judaism and influenced the world. 6 x 9, 240 pp, HC, 978-1-58023-457-3 **$24.99**

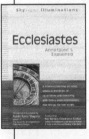

Ecclesiastes: Annotated & Explained
Translation and Annotation by Rabbi Rami Shapiro; Foreword by Rev. Barbara Cawthorne Crafton
5½ x 8½, 160 pp, Quality PB, 978-1-59473-287-4 **$16.99**

Ethics of the Sages: *Pirke Avot*—Annotated & Explained *Translation and Annotation by Rabbi Rami Shapiro* 5½ x 8½, 192 pp, Quality PB, 978-1-59473-207-2 **$16.99**

The Genesis of Leadership: What the Bible Teaches Us about Vision, Values and Leading Change *By Rabbi Nathan Laufer; Foreword by Senator Joseph I. Lieberman*
6 x 9, 288 pp, Quality PB, 978-1-58023-352-1 **$18.99**

Hineini in Our Lives: Learning How to Respond to Others through 14 Biblical Texts and Personal Stories *By Rabbi Norman J. Cohen, PhD* 6 x 9, 240 pp, Quality PB, 978-1-58023-274-6 **$16.99**

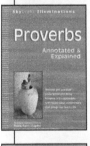

A Man's Responsibility: A Jewish Guide to Being a Son, a Partner in Marriage, a Father and a Community Leader *By Rabbi Joseph B. Meszler* 6 x 9, 192 pp, Quality PB, 978-1-58023-435-1 **$16.99**

The Modern Men's Torah Commentary: New Insights from Jewish Men on the 54 Weekly Torah Portions *Edited by Rabbi Jeffrey K. Salkin*
6 x 9, 368 pp, HC, 978-1-58023-395-8 **$24.99**

Moses and the Journey to Leadership: Timeless Lessons of Effective Management from the Bible and Today's Leaders *By Rabbi Norman J. Cohen, PhD*
6 x 9, 240 pp, Quality PB, 978-1-58023-351-4 **$18.99**; HC, 978-1-58023-227-2 **$21.99**

Proverbs: Annotated & Explained
Translation and Annotation by Rabbi Rami Shapiro
5½ x 8½, 288 pp, Quality PB, 978-1-59473-310-9 **$16.99**

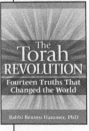

Righteous Gentiles in the Hebrew Bible: Ancient Role Models for Sacred Relationships
By Rabbi Jeffrey K. Salkin; Foreword by Rabbi Harold M. Schulweis;
Preface by Phyllis Tickle 6 x 9, 192 pp, Quality PB, 978-1-58023-364-4 **$18.99**

Sage Tales: Wisdom and Wonder from the Rabbis of the Talmud
By Rabbi Burton L. Visotzky 6 x 9, 256 pp, HC, 978-1-58023-456-6 **$24.99**

The Wisdom of Judaism: An Introduction to the Values of the Talmud
By Rabbi Dov Peretz Elkins 6 x 9, 192 pp, Quality PB, 978-1-58023-327-9 **$16.99**

Or phone, fax, mail or e-mail to: **JEWISH LIGHTS** Publishing
Sunset Farm Offices, Route 4 • P.O. Box 237 • Woodstock, Vermont 05091
Tel: (802) 457-4000 • Fax: (802) 457-4004 • www.jewishlights.com
Credit card orders: **(800) 962-4544** (8:30AM–5:30PM EST Monday–Friday)
Generous discounts on quantity orders. SATISFACTION GUARANTEED. Prices subject to change.

Bar/Bat Mitzvah

The Mitzvah Project Book
Making Mitzvah Part of Your Bar/Bat Mitzvah ... and Your Life
By Liz Suneby and Diane Heiman; Foreword by Rabbi Jeffrey K. Salkin; Preface by Rabbi Sharon Brous
The go-to source for Jewish young adults and their families looking to make the world a better place through good deeds—big or small.
6 x 9, 224 pp, Quality PB Original, 978-1-58023-458-0 **$16.99** For ages 11–13

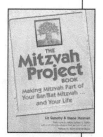

The Bar/Bat Mitzvah Memory Book, 2nd Edition: An Album for Treasuring the Spiritual Celebration
By Rabbi Jeffrey K. Salkin and Nina Salkin
8 x 10, 48 pp, 2-color text, Deluxe HC, ribbon marker, 978-1-58023-263-0 **$19.99**

For Kids—Putting God on Your Guest List, 2nd Edition: How to Claim the Spiritual Meaning of Your Bar or Bat Mitzvah   *By Rabbi Jeffrey K. Salkin*
6 x 9, 144 pp, Quality PB, 978-1-58023-308-8 **$15.99** For ages 11–13

The Jewish Prophet: Visionary Words from Moses and Miriam to Henrietta Szold and A. J. Heschel   *By Rabbi Dr. Michael J. Shire*
6½ x 8½, 128 pp, 123 full-color illus., HC, 978-1-58023-168-8 **$14.95**

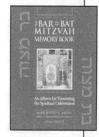

Putting God on the Guest List, 3rd Edition: How to Reclaim the Spiritual Meaning of Your Child's Bar or Bat Mitzvah   *By Rabbi Jeffrey K. Salkin*
6 x 9, 224 pp, Quality PB, 978-1-58023-222-7 **$16.99**; HC, 978-1-58023-260-9 **$24.99**

Putting God on the Guest List Teacher's Guide
8½ x 11, 48 pp, PB, 978-1-58023-226-5 **$8.99**

Teens / Young Adults

Text Messages: A Torah Commentary for Teens
Edited by Rabbi Jeffrey K. Salkin
Shows today's teens how each Torah portion contains worlds of meaning for them, for what they are going through in their lives, and how they can shape their Jewish identity as they enter adulthood.
6 x 9, 304 pp (est), HC, 978-1-58023-507-5 **$24.99**

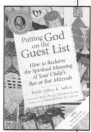

Hannah Senesh: Her Life and Diary, the First Complete Edition
By Hannah Senesh; Foreword by Marge Piercy; Preface by Eitan Senesh; Afterword by Roberta Grossman
6 x 9, 368 pp, b/w photos, Quality PB, 978-1-58023-342-2 **$19.99**

I Am Jewish: Personal Reflections Inspired by the Last Words of Daniel Pearl
Edited by Judea and Ruth Pearl   6 x 9, 304 pp, Deluxe PB w/ flaps, 978-1-58023-259-3 $18.99
Download a free copy of the *I Am Jewish Teacher's Guide* at www.jewishlights.com.

The JGirl's Guide: The Young Jewish Woman's Handbook for Coming of Age
By Penina Adelman, Ali Feldman and Shulamit Reinharz
6 x 9, 240 pp, Quality PB, 978-1-58023-215-9 **$14.99** For ages 11 & up

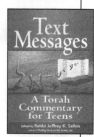

The JGirl's Teacher's and Parent's Guide
8½ x 11, 56 pp, PB, 978-1-58023-225-8 **$8.99**

Tough Questions Jews Ask, 2nd Edition: A Young Adult's Guide to Building a Jewish Life   *By Rabbi Edward Feinstein*
6 x 9, 160 pp, Quality PB, 978-1-58023-454-2 **$16.99** For ages 11 & up

Tough Questions Jews Ask Teacher's Guide
8½ x 11, 72 pp, PB, 978-1-58023-187-9 **$8.95**

Pre-Teens

Be Like God: God's To-Do List for Kids
By Dr. Ron Wolfson
Encourages kids ages eight through twelve to use their God-given superpowers to find the many ways they can make a difference in the lives of others and find meaning and purpose for their own.
7 x 9, 144 pp, Quality PB, 978-1-58023-510-5 **$15.99** For ages 8–12

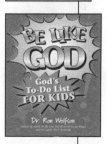

The Book of Miracles: A Young Person's Guide to Jewish Spiritual Awareness
By Lawrence Kushner, with all-new illustrations by the author.
6 x 9, 96 pp, 2-color illus., HC, 978-1-879045-78-1 **$16.95** For ages 9–13

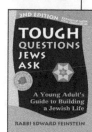

Congregation Resources

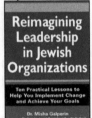

A Practical Guide to Rabbinic Counseling
Edited by Rabbi Yisrael N. Levitz, PhD, and Rabbi Abraham J. Twerski, MD
Provides rabbis with the requisite knowledge and practical guidelines for some of the most common counseling situations.
6 x 9, 432 pp, HC, 978-1-58023-562-4 **$40.00**

Professional Spiritual & Pastoral Care: A Practical Clergy and Chaplain's Handbook
Edited by Rabbi Stephen B. Roberts, MBA, MHL, BCJC
An essential resource integrating the classic foundations of pastoral care with the latest approaches to spiritual care, specifically intended for professionals who work or spend time with congregants in acute care hospitals, behavioral health facilities, rehabilitation centers and long-term care facilities.
6 x 9, 480 pp, HC, 978-1-59473-312-3 **$50.00**

Reimagining Leadership in Jewish Organizations: Ten Practical Lessons to Help You Implement Change and Achieve Your Goals
By Dr. Misha Galperin
Serves as a practical guidepost for lay and professional leaders to evaluate the current paradigm with insights from the world of business, psychology and research in Jewish demographics and sociology. Supported by vignettes from the field that illustrate the successes of the lessons as well as the consequences of not implementing them.
6 x 9, 192 pp, Quality PB, 978-1-58023-492-4 **$16.99**

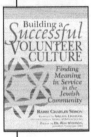

Empowered Judaism: What Independent Minyanim Can Teach Us about Building Vibrant Jewish Communities
By Rabbi Elie Kaunfer; Foreword by Prof. Jonathan D. Sarna
6 x 9, 224 pp, Quality PB, 978-1-58023-412-2 **$18.99**

Building a Successful Volunteer Culture: Finding Meaning in Service in the Jewish Community *By Rabbi Charles Simon; Foreword by Shelley Lindauer; Preface by Dr. Ron Wolfson*
6 x 9, 192 pp, Quality PB, 978-1-58023-408-5 **$16.99**

The Case for Jewish Peoplehood: Can We Be One?
By Dr. Erica Brown and Dr. Misha Galperin; Foreword by Rabbi Joseph Telushkin
6 x 9, 224 pp, HC, 978-1-58023-401-6 **$21.99**

Finding a Spiritual Home: How a New Generation of Jews Can Transform the American Synagogue *By Rabbi Sidney Schwarz*
6 x 9, 352 pp, Quality PB, 978-1-58023-185-5 **$19.95**

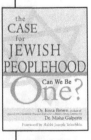

Inspired Jewish Leadership: Practical Approaches to Building Strong Communities
By Dr. Erica Brown 6 x 9, 256 pp, HC, 978-1-58023-361-3 **$27.99**

Jewish Pastoral Care, 2nd Edition: A Practical Handbook from Traditional & Contemporary Sources *Edited by Rabbi Dayle A. Friedman, MSW, MAJCS, BCC*
6 x 9, 528 pp, Quality PB, 978-1-58023-427-6 **$30.00**

Jewish Spiritual Direction: An Innovative Guide from Traditional and Contemporary Sources
Edited by Rabbi Howard A. Addison, PhD, and Barbara Eve Breitman, MSW
6 x 9, 368 pp, HC, 978-1-58023-230-2 **$30.00**

Rethinking Synagogues: A New Vocabulary for Congregational Life
By Rabbi Lawrence A. Hoffman, PhD 6 x 9, 240 pp, Quality PB, 978-1-58023-248-7 **$19.99**

Spiritual Community: The Power to Restore Hope, Commitment and Joy
By Rabbi David A. Teutsch, PhD
5½ x 8½, 144 pp, HC, 978-1-58023-270-8 **$19.99**

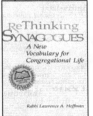

Spiritual Boredom: Rediscovering the Wonder of Judaism *By Dr. Erica Brown*
6 x 9, 208 pp, HC, 978-1-58023-405-4 **$21.99**

The Spirituality of Welcoming: How to Transform Your Congregation into a Sacred Community *By Dr. Ron Wolfson* 6 x 9, 224 pp, Quality PB, 978-1-58023-244-9 **$19.99**

Children's Books

Around the World in One Shabbat
Jewish People Celebrate the Sabbath Together
By Durga Yael Bernhard
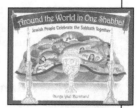
Takes your child on a colorful adventure to share the many ways Jewish people celebrate Shabbat around the world.
11 x 8½, 32 pp, Full-color illus., HC, 978-1-58023-433-7 **$18.99** *For ages 3–6*

It's a … It's a … It's a Mitzvah
By Liz Suneby and Diane Heiman; Full-color Illus. by Laurel Molk
Join Mitzvah Meerkat and friends as they introduce children to the everyday kindnesses that mark the beginning of a Jewish journey and a lifetime commitment to *tikkun olam* (repairing the world). 9 x 12, 32 pp, Full-color illus., HC, 978-1-58023-509-9 **$18.99** *For ages 3–6*
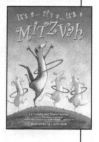

What You Will See Inside a Synagogue
By Rabbi Lawrence A. Hoffman, PhD, and Dr. Ron Wolfson; Full-color photos by Bill Aron
A colorful, fun-to-read introduction that explains the ways and whys of Jewish worship and religious life. 8½ x 10¼, 32 pp, Full-color photos, Quality PB, 978-1-59473-256-0 **$8.99** *For ages 6 & up*
(A book from SkyLight Paths, Jewish Lights' sister imprint)

Because Nothing Looks Like God
By Lawrence Kushner and Karen Kushner
Real-life examples of happiness and sadness—from goodnight stories, to the hope and fear felt the first time at bat, to the closing moments of someone's life—invite parents and children to explore, together, the questions we all have about God, no matter what our age. 11 x 8½, 32 pp, Full-color illus., HC, 978-1-58023-092-6 **$18.99** *For ages 4 & up*

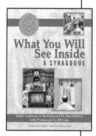

The Book of Miracles: A Young Person's Guide to Jewish Spiritual Awareness
Written and illus. by Lawrence Kushner
Easy-to-read, imaginatively illustrated book encourages kids' awareness of their own spirituality. Revealing the essence of Judaism in a language they can understand and enjoy. 6 x 9, 96 pp, 2-color illus., HC, 978-1-879045-78-1 **$16.95** *For ages 9–13*

In God's Hands   *By Lawrence Kushner and Gary Schmidt*
Brings new life to a traditional Jewish folktale, reminding parents and kids of all faiths and all backgrounds that each of us has the power to make the world a better place—working ordinary miracles with our everyday deeds.
9 x 12, 32 pp, Full-color illus., HC, 978-1-58023-224-1 **$16.99** For ages 5 & up
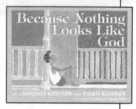

In Our Image: God's First Creatures
By Nancy Sohn Swartz
A playful new twist to the Genesis story, God asks all of nature to offer gifts to humankind—with a promise that the humans would care for creation in return. 9 x 12, 32 pp, Full-color illus., HC, 978-1-879045-99-6 **$16.95** *For ages 4 & up*

The Jewish Family Fun Book, 2nd Ed.
Holiday Projects, Everyday Activities, and Travel Ideas with Jewish Themes
By Danielle Dardashti and Roni Sarig
The complete sourcebook for families wanting to put a new spin on activities for Jewish holidays, holy days and the everyday. It offers dozens of easy-to-do activities that bring Jewish tradition to life for kids of all ages.
6 x 9, 304 pp, w/ 70+ b/w illus., Quality PB, 978-1-58023-333-0 **$18.99**
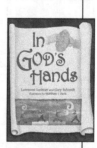

The Kids' Fun Book of Jewish Time   *By Emily Sper*
A unique way to introduce children to the Jewish calendar—night and day, the seven-day week, Shabbat, the Hebrew months, seasons and dates.
9 x 7½, 24 pp, Full-color illus., HC, 978-1-58023-311-8 **$16.99** *For ages 3–6*

What Makes Someone a Jew?   *By Lauren Seidman*
Reflects the changing face of American Judaism. Helps preschoolers and young readers (ages 3–6) understand that you don't have to look a certain way to be Jewish. 10 x 8½, 32 pp, Full-color photos, Quality PB, 978-1-58023-321-7 **$8.99** *For ages 3–6*
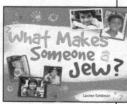

When a Grandparent Dies: A Kid's Own Remembering Workbook for Dealing
with Shiva and the Year Beyond   *By Nechama Liss-Levinson*
8 x 10, 48 pp, 2-color text, HC, 978-1-879045-44-6 **$15.95** *For ages 7–13*

Children's Books by Sandy Eisenberg Sasso

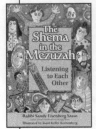

The *Shema* in the Mezuzah: Listening to Each Other
By Sandy Eisenberg Sasso; Full-color Illus. by Joani Keller Rothenberg
This playful yet profound story of conflict and compromise introduces children ages 3 to 6 to the words of the *Shema* and the custom of putting up the mezuzah.
9 x 12, 32 pp, Full-color illus., HC, 978-1-58023-506-8 **$18.99**

Adam & Eve's First Sunset: God's New Day
Explores fear and hope, faith and gratitude in ways that will delight kids and adults—inspiring us to bless each of God's days and nights.
9 x 12, 32 pp, Full-color illus., HC, 978-1-58023-177-0 **$17.95** *For ages 4 & up*

Also Available as a Board Book: **Adam and Eve's New Day**
5 x 5, 24 pp, Full-color illus., Board Book, 978-1-59473-205-8 **$7.99** *For ages 0–4*
(A book from SkyLight Paths, Jewish Lights' sister imprint)

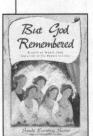

But God Remembered: Stories of Women from Creation to the Promised Land
Four different stories of women—Lilith, Serach, Bityah and the Daughters of Z—teach us important values through their faith and actions.
9 x 12, 32 pp, Full-color illus., Quality PB, 978-1-58023-372-9 **$8.99** *For ages 8 & up*

For Heaven's Sake
Heaven is often found where you least expect it.
9 x 12, 32 pp, Full-color illus., HC, 978-1-58023-054-4 **$16.95** *For ages 4 & up*

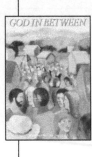

God in Between
If you wanted to find God, where would you look? This magical, mythical tale teaches that God can be found where we are: within all of us and the relationships between us. 9 x 12, 32 pp, Full-color illus., HC, 978-1-879045-86-6 **$16.95** *For ages 4 & up*

God Said Amen
An inspiring story about hearing the answers to our prayers.
9 x 12, 32 pp, Full-color illus., HC, 978-1-58023-080-3 **$16.95** *For ages 4 & up*

God's Paintbrush: Special 10th Anniversary Edition
Wonderfully interactive, invites children of all faiths and backgrounds to encounter God through moments in their own lives. Provides questions adult and child can explore together. 11 x 8½, 32 pp, Full-color illus., HC, 978-1-58023-195-4 **$17.95** *For ages 4 & up*

Also Available as a Board Book: **I Am God's Paintbrush**
5 x 5, 24 pp, Full-color illus., Board Book, 978-1-59473-265-2 **$7.99** *For ages 0–4*
(A book from SkyLight Paths, Jewish Lights' sister imprint)

Also Available: **God's Paintbrush Teacher's Guide**
8½ x 11, 32 pp, PB, 978-1-879045-57-6 **$8.95**

God's Paintbrush Celebration Kit
A Spiritual Activity Kit for Teachers and Students of All Faiths, All Backgrounds
9½ x 12, 40 Full-color Activity Sheets & Teacher Folder w/ complete instructions
HC, 978-1-58023-050-6 **$21.95**
8-Student Activity Sheet Pack (40 sheets/5 sessions), 978-1-58023-058-2 **$19.95**

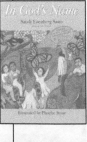

In God's Name
Like an ancient myth in its poetic text and vibrant illustrations, this award-winning modern fable about the search for God's name celebrates the diversity and, at the same time, the unity of all people.
9 x 12, 32 pp, Full-color illus., HC, 978-1-879045-26-2 **$16.99** *For ages 4 & up*

Also Available as a Board Book: **What Is God's Name?**
5 x 5, 24 pp, Full-color illus., Board Book, 978-1-893361-10-2 **$7.99** *For ages 0–4*
(A book from SkyLight Paths, Jewish Lights' sister imprint)

Also Available in Spanish: **El nombre de Dios**
9 x 12, 32 pp, Full-color illus., HC, 978-1-893361-63-8 **$16.95** *For ages 4 & up*

Noah's Wife: The Story of Naamah
9 x 12, 32 pp, Full-color illus., HC, 978-1-58023-134-3 **$16.95** *For ages 4 & up*

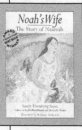

Also Available as a Board Book: **Naamah, Noah's Wife**
5 x 5, 24 pp, Full-color illus., Board Book, 978-1-893361-56-0 **$7.95** *For ages 0–4*
(A book from SkyLight Paths, Jewish Lights' sister imprint)

Ecology/Environment

A Wild Faith: Jewish Ways into Wilderness, Wilderness Ways into Judaism
By Rabbi Mike Comins; Foreword by Nigel Savage 6 x 9, 240 pp, Quality PB, 978-1-58023-316-3 **$16.99**

Ecology & the Jewish Spirit: Where Nature & the Sacred Meet
Edited by Ellen Bernstein 6 x 9, 288 pp, Quality PB, 978-1-58023-082-7 **$18.99**

Torah of the Earth: Exploring 4,000 Years of Ecology in Jewish Thought
Vol. 1: Biblical Israel & Rabbinic Judaism; Vol. 2: Zionism & Eco-Judaism
Edited by Rabbi Arthur Waskow Vol. 1: 6 x 9, 272 pp, Quality PB, 978-1-58023-086-5 **$19.95**
Vol. 2: 6 x 9, 336 pp, Quality PB, 978-1-58023-087-2 **$19.95**

The Way Into Judaism and the Environment *By Jeremy Benstein, PhD*
6 x 9, 288 pp, Quality PB, 978-1-58023-368-2 **$18.99**; HC, 978-1-58023-268-5 **$24.99**

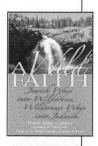

Graphic Novels/Graphic History

The Adventures of Rabbi Harvey: A Graphic Novel of Jewish Wisdom and Wit in the
Wild West *By Steve Sheinkin* 6 x 9, 144 pp, Full-color illus., Quality PB, 978-1-58023-310-1 **$16.99**

Rabbi Harvey Rides Again: A Graphic Novel of Jewish Folktales Let Loose in the
Wild West *By Steve Sheinkin* 6 x 9, 144 pp, Full-color illus., Quality PB, 978-1-58023-347-7 **$16.99**

Rabbi Harvey vs. the Wisdom Kid: A Graphic Novel of Dueling
Jewish Folktales in the Wild West *By Steve Sheinkin*
Rabbi Harvey's first book-length adventure—and toughest challenge.
6 x 9, 144 pp, Full-color illus., Quality PB, 978-1-58023-422-1 **$16.99**

The Story of the Jews: A 4,000-Year Adventure—A Graphic History Book
By Stan Mack 6 x 9, 288 pp, Illus., Quality PB, 978-1-58023-155-8 **$16.99**

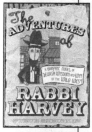

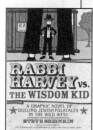

Grief/Healing

Facing Illness, Finding God: How Judaism Can Help You and
Caregivers Cope When Body or Spirit Fails *By Rabbi Joseph B. Meszler*
Will help you find spiritual strength for healing amid the fear, pain and chaos of
illness. 6 x 9, 208 pp, Quality PB, 978-1-58023-423-8 **$16.99**

Midrash & Medicine: Healing Body and Soul in the Jewish Interpretive
Tradition *Edited by Rabbi William Cutter, PhD; Foreword by Michele F. Prince, LCSW, MAJCS*
Explores how midrash can help you see beyond the physical aspects of healing to
tune in to your spiritual source.
6 x 9, 352 pp, Quality PB, 978-1-58023-484-9 **$21.99**

Healing from Despair: Choosing Wholeness in a Broken World
By Rabbi Elie Kaplan Spitz with Erica Shapiro Taylor; Foreword by Abraham J. Twerski, MD
5½ x 8½, 208 pp, Quality PB, 978-1-58023-436-8 **$16.99**

Healing and the Jewish Imagination: Spiritual and Practical Perspectives on
Judaism and Health *Edited by Rabbi William Cutter, PhD*
6 x 9, 240 pp, Quality PB, 978-1-58023-373-6 **$19.99**

Grief in Our Seasons: A Mourner's Kaddish Companion *By Rabbi Kerry M. Olitzky*
4½ x 6½, 448 pp, Quality PB, 978-1-879045-55-2 **$15.95**

Healing of Soul, Healing of Body: Spiritual Leaders Unfold the Strength & Solace
in Psalms *Edited by Rabbi Simkha Y. Weintraub, LCSW*
6 x 9, 128 pp, 2-color illus. text, Quality PB, 978-1-879045-31-6 **$16.99**

Mourning & Mitzvah, 2nd Edition: A Guided Journal for Walking the Mourner's
Path through Grief to Healing *By Rabbi Anne Brener, LCSW*
7½ x 9, 304 pp, Quality PB, 978-1-58023-113-8 **$19.99**

Tears of Sorrow, Seeds of Hope, 2nd Edition: A Jewish Spiritual Companion for
Infertility and Pregnancy Loss *By Rabbi Nina Beth Cardin*
6 x 9, 208 pp, Quality PB, 978-1-58023-233-3 **$18.99**

A Time to Mourn, a Time to Comfort, 2nd Edition: A Guide to Jewish
Bereavement *By Dr. Ron Wolfson; Foreword by Rabbi David J. Wolpe*
7 x 9, 384 pp, Quality PB, 978-1-58023-253-1 **$21.99**

When a Grandparent Dies: A Kid's Own Remembering Workbook for Dealing
with Shiva and the Year Beyond *By Nechama Liss-Levinson, PhD*
8 x 10, 48 pp, 2-color text, HC, 978-1-879045-44-6 **$15.95** *For ages 7–13*

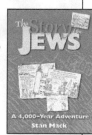

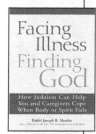

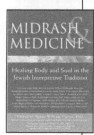

Holidays/Holy Days

Prayers of Awe Series

An exciting new series that examines the High Holy Day liturgy to enrich the praying experience of everyone—whether experienced worshipers or guests who encounter Jewish prayer for the very first time.

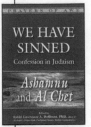

We Have Sinned—Confession in Judaism: *Ashamnu* and *Al Chet*
Edited by Rabbi Lawrence A. Hoffman, PhD
A varied and fascinating look at sin, confession and pardon in Judaism, as suggested by the centrality of *Ashamnu* and *Al Chet*, two prayers that people know so well, though understand so little.   6 x 9, 250 pp (est), HC, 978-1-58023-612-6 **$24.99**

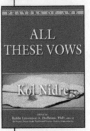

Who by Fire, Who by Water—*Un'taneh Tokef*
Edited by Rabbi Lawrence A. Hoffman, PhD   6 x 9, 272 pp, HC, 978-1-58023-424-5 **$24.99**

All These Vows—*Kol Nidre*
Edited by Rabbi Lawrence A. Hoffman, PhD   6 x 9, 288 pp, HC, 978-1-58023-430-6 **$24.99**

Rosh Hashanah Readings: Inspiration, Information and Contemplation
Yom Kippur Readings: Inspiration, Information and Contemplation
Edited by Rabbi Dov Peretz Elkins; Section Introductions from Arthur Green's These Are the Words
Rosh Hashanah: 6 x 9, 400 pp, Quality PB, 978-1-58023-437-5 **$19.99**
Yom Kippur: 6 x 9, 368 pp, Quality PB, 978-1-58023-438-2 **$19.99**; HC, 978-1-58023-271-5 **$24.99**

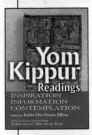

Reclaiming Judaism as a Spiritual Practice: Holy Days and Shabbat
By Rabbi Goldie Milgram   7 x 9, 272 pp, Quality PB, 978-1-58023-205-0 **$19.99**

The Sabbath Soul: Mystical Reflections on the Transformative Power of Holy Time
Selection, Translation and Commentary by Eitan Fishbane, PhD
6 x 9, 208 pp, Quality PB, 978-1-58023-459-7 **$18.99**

Shabbat, 2nd Edition: The Family Guide to Preparing for and Celebrating the Sabbath
By Dr. Ron Wolfson   7 x 9, 320 pp, Illus., Quality PB, 978-1-58023-164-0 **$19.99**

Hanukkah, 2nd Edition: The Family Guide to Spiritual Celebration
By Dr. Ron Wolfson   7 x 9, 240 pp, Illus., Quality PB, 978-1-58023-122-0 **$18.95**

Passover

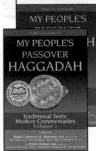

My People's Passover Haggadah
Traditional Texts, Modern Commentaries
Edited by Rabbi Lawrence A. Hoffman, PhD, and David Arnow, PhD
A diverse and exciting collection of commentaries on the traditional Passover Haggadah—in two volumes!
Vol. 1: 7 x 10, 304 pp, HC, 978-1-58023-354-5 **$24.99**
Vol. 2: 7 x 10, 320 pp, HC, 978-1-58023-346-0 **$24.99**

Freedom Journeys: The Tale of Exodus and Wilderness across Millennia
By Rabbi Arthur O. Waskow and Rabbi Phyllis O. Berman
Explores how the story of Exodus echoes in our own time, calling us to relearn and rethink the Passover story through social-justice, ecological, feminist and interfaith perspectives.   6 x 9, 288 pp, HC, 978-1-58023-445-0 **$24.99**

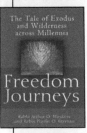

Leading the Passover Journey: The Seder's Meaning Revealed,
the Haggadah's Story Retold   *By Rabbi Nathan Laufer*
Uncovers the hidden meaning of the Seder's rituals and customs.
6 x 9, 224 pp, Quality PB, 978-1-58023-399-6 **$18.99**

Creating Lively Passover Seders, 2nd Edition: A Sourcebook of Engaging Tales,
Texts & Activities   *By David Arnow, PhD*   7 x 9, 464 pp, Quality PB, 978-1-58023-444-3 **$24.99**

Passover, 2nd Edition: The Family Guide to Spiritual Celebration
By Dr. Ron Wolfson with Joel Lurie Grishaver   7 x 9, 416 pp, Quality PB, 978-1-58023-174-9 **$19.95**

The Women's Passover Companion: Women's Reflections on the Festival of Freedom
Edited by Rabbi Sharon Cohen Anisfeld, Tara Mohr and Catherine Spector; Foreword by Paula E. Hyman
6 x 9, 352 pp, Quality PB, 978-1-58023-231-9 **$19.99**; HC, 978-1-58023-128-2 **$24.95**

The Women's Seder Sourcebook: Rituals & Readings for Use at the Passover Seder
Edited by Rabbi Sharon Cohen Anisfeld, Tara Mohr and Catherine Spector
6 x 9, 384 pp, Quality PB, 978-1-58023-232-6 **$19.99**

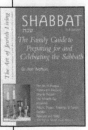
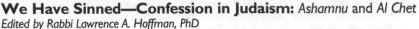

Inspiration

God of Me: Imagining God throughout Your Lifetime
By Rabbi David Lyon Helps you cut through preconceived ideas of God and dogmas that stifle your creativity when thinking about your personal relationship with God. 6 x 9, 176 pp, Quality PB, 978-1-58023-452-8 **$16.99**

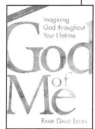

The God Upgrade: Finding Your 21st-Century Spirituality in Judaism's 5,000-Year-Old Tradition *By Rabbi Jamie Korngold; Foreword by Rabbi Harold M. Schulweis* A provocative look at how our changing God concepts have shaped every aspect of Judaism. 6 x 9, 176 pp, Quality PB, 978-1-58023-443-6 **$15.99**

The Seven Questions You're Asked in Heaven: Reviewing and Renewing Your Life on Earth *By Dr. Ron Wolfson* An intriguing and entertaining resource for living a life that matters. 6 x 9, 176 pp, Quality PB, 978-1-58023-407-8 **$16.99**

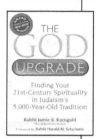

Happiness and the Human Spirit: The Spirituality of Becoming the Best You Can Be *By Rabbi Abraham J. Twerski, MD*
Shows you that true happiness is attainable once you stop looking outside yourself for the source. 6 x 9, 176 pp, Quality PB, 978-1-58023-404-7 **$16.99**; HC, 978-1-58023-343-9 **$19.99**

A Formula for Proper Living: Practical Lessons from Life and Torah
By Rabbi Abraham J. Twerski, MD 6 x 9, 144 pp, HC, 978-1-58023-402-3 **$19.99**

The Bridge to Forgiveness: Stories and Prayers for Finding God and Restoring Wholeness *By Rabbi Karyn D. Kedar* 6 x 9, 176 pp, Quality PB, 978-1-58023-451-1 **$16.99**

The Empty Chair: Finding Hope and Joy—Timeless Wisdom from a Hasidic Master, Rebbe Nachman of Breslov *Adapted by Moshe Mykoff and the Breslov Research Institute* 4 x 6, 128 pp, Deluxe PB w/ flaps, 978-1-879045-67-5 **$9.99**

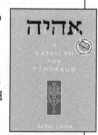

The Gentle Weapon: Prayers for Everyday and Not-So-Everyday Moments— Timeless Wisdom from the Teachings of the Hasidic Master, Rebbe Nachman of Breslov *Adapted by Moshe Mykoff and S. C. Mizrahi, together with the Breslov Research Institute* 4 x 6, 144 pp, Deluxe PB w/ flaps, 978-1-58023-022-3 **$9.99**

God Whispers: Stories of the Soul, Lessons of the Heart *By Rabbi Karyn D. Kedar* 6 x 9, 176 pp, Quality PB, 978-1-58023-088-9 **$15.95**

God's To-Do List: 103 Ways to Be an Angel and Do God's Work on Earth
By Dr. Ron Wolfson 6 x 9, 144 pp, Quality PB, 978-1-58023-301-9 **$16.99**

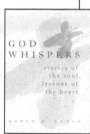

Jewish Stories from Heaven and Earth: Inspiring Tales to Nourish the Heart and Soul *Edited by Rabbi Dov Peretz Elkins* 6 x 9, 304 pp, Quality PB, 978-1-58023-363-7 **$16.99**

Life's Daily Blessings: Inspiring Reflections on Gratitude and Joy for Every Day, Based on Jewish Wisdom *By Rabbi Kerry M. Olitzky* 4½ x 6½, 368 pp, Quality PB, 978-1-58023-396-5 **$16.99**

Restful Reflections: Nighttime Inspiration to Calm the Soul, Based on Jewish Wisdom *By Rabbi Kerry M. Olitzky and Rabbi Lori Forman-Jacobi* 4½ x 6½, 448 pp, Quality PB, 978-1-58023-091-9 **$16.99**

Sacred Intentions: Morning Inspiration to Strengthen the Spirit, Based on Jewish Wisdom *By Rabbi Kerry M. Olitzky and Rabbi Lori Forman-Jacobi* 4½ x 6½, 448 pp, Quality PB, 978-1-58023-061-2 **$16.99**

Kabbalah/Mysticism

Jewish Mysticism and the Spiritual Life: Classical Texts, Contemporary Reflections *Edited by Dr. Lawrence Fine, Dr. Eitan Fishbane and Rabbi Or N. Rose* Inspirational and thought-provoking materials for contemplation, discussion and action. 6 x 9, 256 pp, HC, 978-1-58023-434-4 **$24.99**

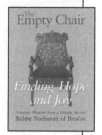

Ehyeh: A Kabbalah for Tomorrow
By Rabbi Arthur Green, PhD 6 x 9, 224 pp, Quality PB, 978-1-58023-213-5 **$18.99**

The Gift of Kabbalah: Discovering the Secrets of Heaven, Renewing Your Life on Earth
By Tamar Frankiel, PhD 6 x 9, 256 pp, Quality PB, 978-1-58023-141-1 **$16.95**

Seek My Face: A Jewish Mystical Theology *By Rabbi Arthur Green, PhD*
6 x 9, 304 pp, Quality PB, 978-1-58023-130-5 **$19.95**

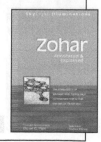

Zohar: Annotated & Explained *Translation & Annotation by Dr. Daniel C. Matt; Foreword by Andrew Harvey* 5½ x 8½, 176 pp, Quality PB, 978-1-893361-51-5 **$15.99**
(A book from SkyLight Paths, Jewish Lights' sister imprint)

See also *The Way Into Jewish Mystical Tradition* in The Way Into... Series.

Life Cycle
Marriage/Parenting/Family/Aging

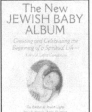

The New Jewish Baby Album: Creating and Celebrating the Beginning of a Spiritual Life—A Jewish Lights Companion
By the Editors at Jewish Lights; Foreword by Anita Diamant; Preface by Rabbi Sandy Eisenberg Sasso
A spiritual keepsake that will be treasured for generations. More than just a memory book, *shows you how—and why it's important*—to create a Jewish home and a Jewish life. 8 x 10, 64 pp, Deluxe Padded HC, Full-color illus., 978-1-58023-138-1 **$19.95**

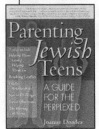

The Jewish Pregnancy Book: A Resource for the Soul, Body & Mind during Pregnancy, Birth & the First Three Months By Sandy Falk, MD, and Rabbi Daniel Judson, with Steven A. Rapp Medical information, prayers and rituals for each stage of pregnancy. 7 x 10, 208 pp, b/w photos, Quality PB, 978-1-58023-178-7 **$16.95**

Celebrating Your New Jewish Daughter: Creating Jewish Ways to Welcome Baby Girls into the Covenant—New and Traditional Ceremonies By Debra Nussbaum Cohen; Foreword by Rabbi Sandy Eisenberg Sasso 6 x 9, 272 pp, Quality PB, 978-1-58023-090-2 **$18.95**

The New Jewish Baby Book, 2nd Edition: Names, Ceremonies & Customs—A Guide for Today's Families By Anita Diamant 6 x 9, 320 pp, Quality PB, 978-1-58023-251-7 **$19.99**

Parenting as a Spiritual Journey: Deepening Ordinary and Extraordinary Events into Sacred Occasions By Rabbi Nancy Fuchs-Kreimer, PhD
6 x 9, 224 pp, Quality PB, 978-1-58023-016-2 **$17.99**

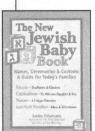

Parenting Jewish Teens: A Guide for the Perplexed
By Joanne Doades Explores the questions and issues that shape the world in which today's Jewish teenagers live and offers constructive advice to parents. 6 x 9, 176 pp, Quality PB, 978-1-58023-305-7 **$16.99**

Judaism for Two: A Spiritual Guide for Strengthening and Celebrating Your Loving Relationship By Rabbi Nancy Fuchs-Kreimer, PhD, and Rabbi Nancy H. Wiener, DMin; Foreword by Rabbi Elliot N. Dorff, PhD
Addresses the ways Jewish teachings can enhance and strengthen committed relationships. 6 x 9, 224 pp, Quality PB, 978-1-58023-254-8 **$16.99**

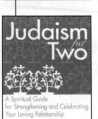

The Creative Jewish Wedding Book, 2nd Edition: A Hands-On Guide to New & Old Traditions, Ceremonies & Celebrations By Gabrielle Kaplan-Mayer 9 x 9, 288 pp, b/w photos, Quality PB, 978-1-58023-398-9 **$19.99**

Divorce Is a Mitzvah: A Practical Guide to Finding Wholeness and Holiness When Your Marriage Dies By Rabbi Perry Netter; Afterword by Rabbi Laura Geller 6 x 9, 224 pp, Quality PB, 978-1-58023-172-5 **$16.95**

Embracing the Covenant: Converts to Judaism Talk About Why & How
By Rabbi Allan Berkowitz and Patti Moskovitz 6 x 9, 192 pp, Quality PB, 978-1-879045-50-7 **$16.95**

The Guide to Jewish Interfaith Family Life: An InterfaithFamily.com Handbook
Edited by Ronnie Friedland and Edmund Case
6 x 9, 384 pp, Quality PB, 978-1-58023-153-4 **$18.95**

A Heart of Wisdom: Making the Jewish Journey from Midlife through the Elder Years
Edited by Susan Berrin; Foreword by Rabbi Harold Kushner
6 x 9, 384 pp, Quality PB, 978-1-58023-051-3 **$18.95**

Introducing My Faith and My Community: The Jewish Outreach Institute Guide for the Christian in a Jewish Interfaith Relationship
By Rabbi Kerry M. Olitzky 6 x 9, 176 pp, Quality PB, 978-1-58023-192-3 **$16.99**

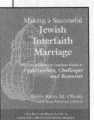

Making a Successful Jewish Interfaith Marriage: The Jewish Outreach Institute Guide to Opportunities, Challenges and Resources By Rabbi Kerry M. Olitzky with Joan Peterson Littman
6 x 9, 176 pp, Quality PB, 978-1-58023-170-1 **$16.95**

A Man's Responsibility: A Jewish Guide to Being a Son, a Partner in Marriage, a Father and a Community Leader By Rabbi Joseph B. Meszler
6 x 9, 192 pp, Quality PB, 978-1-58023-435-1 **$16.99**; HC, 978-1-58023-362-0 **$21.99**

So That Your Values Live On: Ethical Wills and How to Prepare Them
Edited by Rabbi Jack Riemer and Rabbi Nathaniel Stampfer
6 x 9, 272 pp, Quality PB, 978-1-879045-34-7 **$18.99**

Meditation

Jewish Meditation Practices for Everyday Life
Awakening Your Heart, Connecting with God
By Rabbi Jeff Roth
Offers a fresh take on meditation that draws on life experience and living life with greater clarity as opposed to the traditional method of rigorous study.
6 x 9, 224 pp, Quality PB, 978-1-58023-397-2 **$18.99**

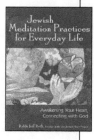

The Handbook of Jewish Meditation Practices
A Guide for Enriching the Sabbath and Other Days of Your Life
By Rabbi David A. Cooper Easy-to-learn meditation techniques.
6 x 9, 208 pp, Quality PB, 978-1-58023-102-2 **$16.95**

Discovering Jewish Meditation, 2nd Edition
Instruction & Guidance for Learning an Ancient Spiritual Practice
By Nan Fink Gefen, PhD 6 x 9, 208 pp, Quality PB, 978-1-58023-462-7 **$16.99**

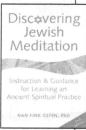

Meditation from the Heart of Judaism
Today's Teachers Share Their Practices, Techniques, and Faith
Edited by Avram Davis 6 x 9, 256 pp, Quality PB, 978-1-58023-049-0 **$16.95**

Ritual/Sacred Practices

The Jewish Dream Book: The Key to Opening the Inner Meaning of Your Dreams *By Vanessa L. Ochs, PhD, with Elizabeth Ochs; Illus. by Kristina Swarner*
Instructions for how modern people can perform ancient Jewish dream practices and dream interpretations drawn from the Jewish wisdom tradition.
8 x 8, 128 pp, Full-color illus., Deluxe PB w/ flaps, 978-1-58023-132-9 **$16.95**

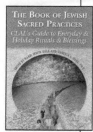

God in Your Body: Kabbalah, Mindfulness and Embodied Spiritual Practice
By Jay Michaelson
The first comprehensive treatment of the body in Jewish spiritual practice and an essential guide to the sacred.
6 x 9, 272 pp, Quality PB, 978-1-58023-304-0 **$18.99**

The Book of Jewish Sacred Practices: CLAL's Guide to Everyday &
Holiday Rituals & Blessings *Edited by Rabbi Irwin Kula and Vanessa L. Ochs, PhD*
6 x 9, 368 pp, Quality PB, 978-1-58023-152-7 **$18.95**

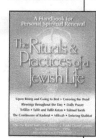

Jewish Ritual: A Brief Introduction for Christians
By Rabbi Kerry M. Olitzky and Rabbi Daniel Judson
5½ x 8½, 144 pp, Quality PB, 978-1-58023-210-4 **$14.99**

The Rituals & Practices of a Jewish Life: A Handbook for Personal Spiritual
Renewal *Edited by Rabbi Kerry M. Olitzky and Rabbi Daniel Judson*
6 x 9, 272 pp, Illus., Quality PB, 978-1-58023-169-5 **$18.95**

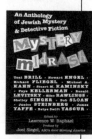

The Sacred Art of Lovingkindness: Preparing to Practice
By Rabbi Rami Shapiro 5½ x 8½, 176 pp, Quality PB, 978-1-59473-151-8 **$16.99**
(A book from SkyLight Paths, Jewish Lights' sister imprint)

Science Fiction/Mystery & Detective Fiction

Criminal Kabbalah: An Intriguing Anthology of Jewish Mystery &
Detective Fiction *Edited by Lawrence W. Raphael; Foreword by Laurie R. King*
All-new stories from twelve of today's masters of mystery and detective fiction—sure to delight mystery buffs of all faith traditions.
6 x 9, 256 pp, Quality PB, 978-1-58023-109-1 **$16.95**

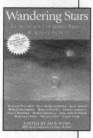

Mystery Midrash: An Anthology of Jewish Mystery & Detective Fiction
Edited by Lawrence W. Raphael; Preface by Joel Siegel
6 x 9, 304 pp, Quality PB, 978-1-58023-055-1 **$16.95**

Wandering Stars: An Anthology of Jewish Fantasy & Science Fiction
Edited by Jack Dann; Introduction by Isaac Asimov
6 x 9, 272 pp, Quality PB, 978-1-58023-005-6 **$18.99**

More Wandering Stars: An Anthology of Outstanding Stories of Jewish Fantasy and
Science Fiction *Edited by Jack Dann; Introduction by Isaac Asimov*
6 x 9, 192 pp, Quality PB, 978-1-58023-063-6 **$16.95**

Social Justice

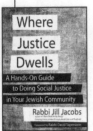

Where Justice Dwells
A Hands-On Guide to Doing Social Justice in Your Jewish Community
By Rabbi Jill Jacobs; Foreword by Rabbi David Saperstein
Provides ways to envision and act on your own ideals of social justice.
7 x 9, 288 pp, Quality PB Original, 978-1-58023-453-5 **$24.99**

There Shall Be No Needy
Pursuing Social Justice through Jewish Law and Tradition
By Rabbi Jill Jacobs; Foreword by Rabbi Elliot N. Dorff, PhD; Preface by Simon Greer
Confronts the most pressing issues of twenty-first-century America from a deeply Jewish perspective. 6 x 9, 288 pp, Quality PB, 978-1-58023-425-2 **$16.99**

There Shall Be No Needy Teacher's Guide 8½ x 11, 56 pp, PB, 978-1-58023-429-0 **$8.99**

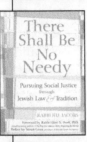

Conscience
The Duty to Obey and the Duty to Disobey
By Rabbi Harold M. Schulweis
Examines the idea of conscience and the role conscience plays in our relationships to government, law, ethics, religion, human nature, God—and to each other.
6 x 9, 160 pp, Quality PB, 978-1-58023-419-1 **$16.99**; HC, 978-1-58023-375-0 **$19.99**

Judaism and Justice
The Jewish Passion to Repair the World
By Rabbi Sidney Schwarz; Foreword by Ruth Messinger
Explores the relationship between Judaism, social justice and the Jewish identity of American Jews. 6 x 9, 352 pp, Quality PB, 978-1-58023-353-8 **$19.99**

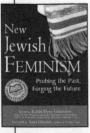

Spirituality/Women's Interest

New Jewish Feminism
Probing the Past, Forging the Future
Edited by Rabbi Elyse Goldstein; Foreword by Anita Diamant
Looks at the growth and accomplishments of Jewish feminism and what they mean for Jewish women today and tomorrow.
6 x 9, 480 pp, HC, 978-1-58023-359-0 **$24.99**

The Divine Feminine in Biblical Wisdom Literature
Selections Annotated & Explained
Translation & Annotation by Rabbi Rami Shapiro
5½ x 8½, 240 pp, Quality PB, 978-1-59473-109-9 **$16.99**
(A book from SkyLight Paths, Jewish Lights' sister imprint)

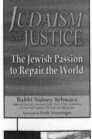

The Quotable Jewish Woman
Wisdom, Inspiration & Humor from the Mind & Heart
Edited by Elaine Bernstein Partnow
6 x 9, 496 pp, Quality PB, 978-1-58023-236-4 **$19.99**

The Women's Haftarah Commentary
New Insights from Women Rabbis on the 54 Weekly Haftarah Portions, the 5 Megillot & Special Shabbatot
Edited by Rabbi Elyse Goldstein
Illuminates the historical significance of female portrayals in the Haftarah and the Five Megillot. 6 x 9, 560 pp, Quality PB, 978-1-58023-371-2 **$19.99**

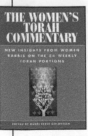

The Women's Torah Commentary
New Insights from Women Rabbis on the 54 Weekly Torah Portions
Edited by Rabbi Elyse Goldstein
Over fifty women rabbis offer inspiring insights on the Torah, in a week-by-week format.
6 x 9, 496 pp, Quality PB, 978-1-58023-370-5 **$19.99**; HC, 978-1-58023-076-6 **$34.95**

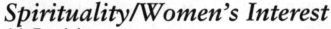

See Passover for *The Women's Passover Companion: Women's Reflections on the Festival of Freedom* and *The Women's Seder Sourcebook: Rituals & Readings for Use at the Passover Seder.*

Spirituality

The Jewish Lights Spirituality Handbook: A Guide to Understanding, Exploring & Living a Spiritual Life *Edited by Stuart M. Matlins*
What exactly is "Jewish" about spirituality? How do I make it a part of my life? Fifty of today's foremost spiritual leaders share their ideas and experience with us.
6 x 9, 456 pp, Quality PB, 978-1-58023-093-3 **$19.99**

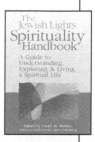

The Sabbath Soul: Mystical Reflections on the Transformative Power of Holy Time *Selection, Translation and Commentary by Eitan Fishbane, PhD*
Explores the writings of mystical masters of Hasidism. Provides translations and interpretations of a wide range of Hasidic sources previously unavailable in English that reflect the spiritual transformation that takes place on the seventh day.
6 x 9, 208 pp, Quality PB, 978-1-58023-459-7 **$18.99**

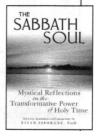

Repentance: The Meaning and Practice of *Teshuvah*
By Dr. Louis E. Newman; Foreword by Rabbi Harold M. Schulweis; Preface by Rabbi Karyn D. Kedar
Examines both the practical and philosophical dimensions of *teshuvah*, Judaism's core religious-moral teaching on repentance, and its value for us—Jews and non-Jews alike—today. 6 x 9, 256 pp, HC, 978-1-58023-426-9 **$24.99**

Aleph-Bet Yoga: Embodying the Hebrew Letters for Physical and Spiritual Well-Being
By Steven A. Rapp; Foreword by Tamar Frankiel, PhD, and Judy Greenfeld; Preface by Hart Lazer
7 x 10, 128 pp, b/w photos, Quality PB, Lay-flat binding, 978-1-58023-162-6 **$16.95**

A Book of Life: Embracing Judaism as a Spiritual Practice
By Rabbi Michael Strassfeld 6 x 9, 544 pp, Quality PB, 978-1-58023-247-0 **$19.99**

Bringing the Psalms to Life: How to Understand and Use the Book of Psalms
By Rabbi Daniel F. Polish, PhD 6 x 9, 208 pp, Quality PB, 978-1-58023-157-2 **$16.95**

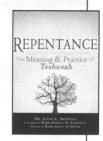

Does the Soul Survive? A Jewish Journey to Belief in Afterlife, Past Lives & Living with Purpose *By Rabbi Elie Kaplan Spitz; Foreword by Brian L. Weiss, MD*
6 x 9, 288 pp, Quality PB, 978-1-58023-165-7 **$16.99**

Entering the Temple of Dreams: Jewish Prayers, Movements and Meditations for the End of the Day *By Tamar Frankiel, PhD, and Judy Greenfeld*
7 x 10, 192 pp, illus., Quality PB, 978-1-58023-079-7 **$16.95**

First Steps to a New Jewish Spirit: Reb Zalman's Guide to Recapturing the Intimacy & Ecstasy in Your Relationship with God *By Rabbi Zalman M. Schachter-Shalomi with Donald Gropman* 6 x 9, 144 pp, Quality PB, 978-1-58023-182-4 **$16.95**

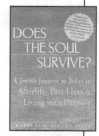

Foundations of Sephardic Spirituality: The Inner Life of Jews of the Ottoman Empire
By Rabbi Marc D. Angel, PhD 6 x 9, 224 pp, Quality PB, 978-1-58023-341-5 **$18.99**

God & the Big Bang: Discovering Harmony between Science & Spirituality
By Dr. Daniel C. Matt 6 x 9, 216 pp, Quality PB, 978-1-879045-89-7 **$18.99**

God in Our Relationships: Spirituality between People from the Teachings of Martin Buber *By Rabbi Dennis S. Ross* 5½ x 8½, 160 pp, Quality PB, 978-1-58023-147-3 **$16.95**

Judaism, Physics and God: Searching for Sacred Metaphors in a Post-Einstein World
By Rabbi David W. Nelson 6 x 9, 352 pp, Quality PB, inc. reader's discussion guide,
978-1-58023-306-4 **$18.99**; HC, 352 pp, 978-1-58023-252-4 **$24.99**

Meaning & Mitzvah: Daily Practices for Reclaiming Judaism through Prayer, God, Torah, Hebrew, Mitzvot and Peoplehood *By Rabbi Goldie Milgram*
7 x 9, 336 pp, Quality PB, 978-1-58023-256-2 **$19.99**

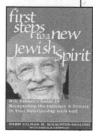

Minding the Temple of the Soul: Balancing Body, Mind, and Spirit through Traditional Jewish Prayer, Movement, and Meditation *By Tamar Frankiel, PhD, and Judy Greenfeld*
7 x 10, 184 pp, illus., Quality PB, 978-1-879045-64-4 **$18.99**

One God Clapping: The Spiritual Path of a Zen Rabbi *By Rabbi Alan Lew with Sherril Jaffe*
5½ x 8½, 336 pp, Quality PB, 978-1-58023-115-2 **$16.95**

The Soul of the Story: Meetings with Remarkable People
By Rabbi David Zeller 6 x 9, 288 pp, HC, 978-1-58023-272-2 **$21.99**

Tanya, the Masterpiece of Hasidic Wisdom: Selections Annotated & Explained
Translation & Annotation by Rabbi Rami Shapiro; Foreword by Rabbi Zalman M. Schachter-Shalomi
5½ x 8½, 240 pp, Quality PB, 978-1-59473-275-1 **$16.99**

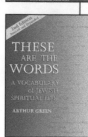

These Are the Words, 2nd Edition: A Vocabulary of Jewish Spiritual Life
By Rabbi Arthur Green, PhD 6 x 9, 320 pp, Quality PB, 978-1-58023-494-8 **$19.99**

Spirituality/Prayer

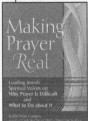

Making Prayer Real: Leading Jewish Spiritual Voices on Why Prayer Is Difficult and What to Do about It *By Rabbi Mike Comins*
A new and different response to the challenges of Jewish prayer, with "best prayer practices" from Jewish spiritual leaders of all denominations.
6 x 9, 320 pp, Quality PB, 978-1-58023-417-7 **$18.99**

Witnesses to the One: The Spiritual History of the *Sh'ma*
By Rabbi Joseph B. Meszler; Foreword by Rabbi Elyse Goldstein
6 x 9, 176 pp, Quality PB, 978-1-58023-400-9 **$16.99**; HC, 978-1-58023-309-5 **$19.99**

My People's Prayer Book Series: Traditional Prayers, Modern Commentaries *Edited by Rabbi Lawrence A. Hoffman, PhD*
Provides diverse and exciting commentary to the traditional liturgy. Will help you find new wisdom in Jewish prayer, and bring liturgy into your life. Each book

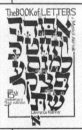

includes Hebrew text, modern translations and commentaries from all perspectives of the Jewish world.
Vol. 1—The *Sh'ma* and Its Blessings
   7 x 10, 168 pp, HC, 978-1-879045-79-8 **$29.99**
Vol. 2—The *Amidah* 7 x 10, 240 pp, HC, 978-1-879045-80-4 **$24.95**
Vol. 3—*P'sukei D'zimrah* (Morning Psalms)
   7 x 10, 240 pp, HC, 978-1-879045-81-1 **$29.99**
Vol. 4—*Seder K'riat Hatorah* (The Torah Service)
   7 x 10, 264 pp, HC, 978-1-879045-82-8 **$29.99**
Vol. 5—*Birkhot Hashachar* (Morning Blessings)
   7 x 10, 240 pp, HC, 978-1-879045-83-5 **$24.95**
Vol. 6—*Tachanun* and Concluding Prayers
   7 x 10, 240 pp, HC, 978-1-879045-84-2 **$24.95**
Vol. 7—Shabbat at Home 7 x 10, 240 pp, HC, 978-1-879045-85-9 **$24.95**
Vol. 8—*Kabbalat Shabbat* (Welcoming Shabbat in the Synagogue)
   7 x 10, 240 pp, HC, 978-1-58023-121-3 **$24.99**
Vol. 9—Welcoming the Night: *Minchah* and *Ma'ariv* (Afternoon and
   Evening Prayer) 7 x 10, 272 pp, HC, 978-1-58023-262-3 **$24.99**
Vol. 10—Shabbat Morning: *Shacharit* and *Musaf* (Morning and
   Additional Services) 7 x 10, 240 pp, HC, 978-1-58023-240-1 **$29.99**

Spirituality/Lawrence Kushner

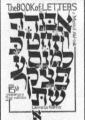

I'm God; You're Not: Observations on Organized Religion & Other Disguises of the Ego
6 x 9, 256 pp, Quality PB, 978-1-58023-513-6 **$18.99**; HC, 978-1-58023-441-2 **$21.99**

The Book of Letters: A Mystical Hebrew Alphabet
Popular HC Edition, 6 x 9, 80 pp, 2-color text, 978-1-879045-00-2 **$24.95**
Collector's Limited Edition, 9 x 12, 80 pp, gold-foil-embossed pages, w/ limited-edition silkscreened print, 978-1-879045-04-0 **$349.00**

The Book of Miracles: A Young Person's Guide to Jewish Spiritual Awareness
6 x 9, 96 pp, 2-color illus., HC, 978-1-879045-78-1 **$16.95** *For ages 9–13*

The Book of Words: Talking Spiritual Life, Living Spiritual Talk
6 x 9, 160 pp, Quality PB, 978-1-58023-020-9 **$18.99**

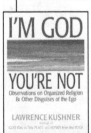

Eyes Remade for Wonder: A Lawrence Kushner Reader *Introduction by Thomas Moore*
6 x 9, 240 pp, Quality PB, 978-1-58023-042-1 **$18.95**

God Was in This Place & I, i Did Not Know: Finding Self, Spirituality and Ultimate Meaning 6 x 9, 192 pp, Quality PB, 978-1-879045-33-0 **$16.95**

Honey from the Rock: An Introduction to Jewish Mysticism
6 x 9, 176 pp, Quality PB, 978-1-58023-073-5 **$16.95**

Invisible Lines of Connection: Sacred Stories of the Ordinary
5½ x 8½, 160 pp, Quality PB, 978-1-879045-98-9 **$15.95**

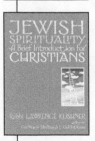

Jewish Spirituality: A Brief Introduction for Christians
5½ x 8½, 112 pp, Quality PB, 978-1-58023-150-3 **$12.95**

The River of Light: Jewish Mystical Awareness
6 x 9, 192 pp, Quality PB, 978-1-58023-096-4 **$16.95**

The Way Into Jewish Mystical Tradition
6 x 9, 224 pp, Quality PB, 978-1-58023-200-5 **$18.99**; HC, 978-1-58023-029-2 **$21.95**

Spirituality/Crafts

Jewish Threads: A Hands-On Guide to Stitching Spiritual Intention into Jewish Fabric Crafts *By Diana Drew with Robert Grayson*
Learn how to make your own Jewish fabric crafts with spiritual intention—a journey of creativity, imagination and inspiration. Thirty projects.
7 x 9, 288 pp, 8-page color insert, b/w illus., Quality PB Original, 978-1-58023-442-9 **$19.99**

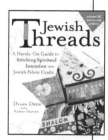

(from SkyLight Paths, Jewish Lights' sister imprint)

Beading—The Creative Spirit: Finding Your Sacred Center through the Art of Beadwork *By Wendy Ellsworth*
Invites you on a spiritual pilgrimage into the kaleidoscope world of glass and color.
7 x 9, 240 pp, 8-page full-color insert, b/w photos and diagrams, Quality PB, 978-1-59473-267-6 **$18.99**

Contemplative Crochet: A Hands-On Guide for Interlocking Faith and Craft *By Cindy Crandall-Frazier; Foreword by Linda Skolnik*
Will take you on a path deeper into your crocheting and your spiritual awareness.
7 x 9, 208 pp, b/w photos, Quality PB, 978-1-59473-238-6 **$16.99**

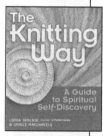

The Knitting Way: A Guide to Spiritual Self-Discovery
By Linda Skolnik and Janice MacDaniels
Shows how to use knitting to strengthen your spiritual self.
7 x 9, 240 pp, b/w photos, Quality PB, 978-1-59473-079-5 **$16.99**

The Painting Path: Embodying Spiritual Discovery through Yoga, Brush and Color *By Linda Novick; Foreword by Richard Segalman*
Explores the divine connection you can experience through art.
7 x 9, 208 pp, 8-page full-color insert, b/w photos, Quality PB, 978-1-59473-226-3 **$18.99**

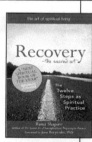

The Quilting Path: A Guide to Spiritual Self-Discovery through Fabric, Thread and Kabbalah *By Louise Silk* Explores how to cultivate personal growth through quilt making. 7 x 9, 192 pp, b/w photos, Quality PB, 978-1-59473-206-5 **$16.99**

The Scrapbooking Journey: A Hands-On Guide to Spiritual Discovery
By Cory Richardson-Lauve; Foreword by Stacy Julian
Reveals how this craft can become a practice used to deepen and shape your life.
7 x 9, 176 pp, 8-page full-color insert, b/w photos, Quality PB, 978-1-59473-216-4 **$18.99**

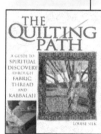

Travel

Israel—A Spiritual Travel Guide, 2nd Edition: A Companion for the Modern Jewish Pilgrim *By Rabbi Lawrence A. Hoffman, PhD*
Helps today's pilgrim tap into the deep spiritual meaning of the ancient—and modern—sites of the Holy Land.
4¾ x 10, 256 pp, Illus., Quality PB, 978-1-58023-261-6 **$18.99**
Also Available: **The Israel Mission Leader's Guide** 5½ x 8½, 16 pp, PB, 978-1-58023-085-8 **$4.95**

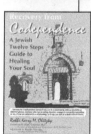

Twelve Steps

Recovery—The Sacred Art: The Twelve Steps as Spiritual Practice
By Rami Shapiro; Foreword by Joan Borysenko, PhD
Draws on insights and practices of different religious traditions to help you move more deeply into the universal spirituality of the Twelve Step system.
5½ x 8½, 240 pp, Quality PB Original, 978-1-59473-259-1 **$16.99**
(A book from SkyLight Paths, Jewish Lights' sister imprint)

100 Blessings Every Day: Daily Twelve Step Recovery Affirmations, Exercises for Personal Growth & Renewal Reflecting Seasons of the Jewish Year *By Rabbi Kerry M. Olitzky; Foreword by Rabbi Neil Gillman, PhD* 4½ x 6½, 432 pp, Quality PB, 978-1-879045-30-9 **$16.99**

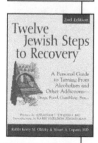

Recovery from Codependence: A Jewish Twelve Steps Guide to Healing Your Soul
By Rabbi Kerry M. Olitzky 6 x 9, 160 pp, Quality PB, 978-1-879045-32-3 **$13.95**

Twelve Jewish Steps to Recovery, 2nd Edition: A Personal Guide to Turning from Alcoholism & Other Addictions—Drugs, Food, Gambling, Sex...
By Rabbi Kerry M. Olitzky and Stuart A. Copans, MD; Preface by Abraham J. Twerski, MD
6 x 9, 160 pp, Quality PB, 978-1-58023-409-2 **$16.99**

Theology/Philosophy/The Way Into... Series

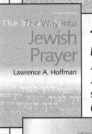

The Way Into... series offers an accessible and highly usable "guided tour" of the Jewish faith, people, history and beliefs—in total, an introduction to Judaism that will enable you to understand and interact with the sacred texts of the Jewish tradition. Each volume is written by a leading contemporary scholar and teacher, and explores one key aspect of Judaism. The Way Into... series enables all readers to achieve a real sense of Jewish cultural literacy through guided study.

The Way Into Encountering God in Judaism
By Rabbi Neil Gillman, PhD
For everyone who wants to understand how Jews have encountered God throughout history and today.
6 x 9, 240 pp, Quality PB, 978-1-58023-199-2 **$18.99**; HC, 978-1-58023-025-4 **$21.95**
Also Available: **The Jewish Approach to God:** A Brief Introduction for Christians
By Rabbi Neil Gillman, PhD
5½ x 8½, 192 pp, Quality PB, 978-1-58023-190-9 **$16.95**

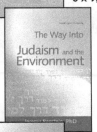

The Way Into Jewish Mystical Tradition
By Rabbi Lawrence Kushner
Allows readers to interact directly with the sacred mystical texts of the Jewish tradition. An accessible introduction to the concepts of Jewish mysticism, their religious and spiritual significance, and how they relate to life today.
6 x 9, 224 pp, Quality PB, 978-1-58023-200-5 **$18.99**; HC, 978-1-58023-029-2 **$21.95**

The Way Into Jewish Prayer
By Rabbi Lawrence A. Hoffman, PhD
Opens the door to 3,000 years of Jewish prayer, making anyone feel at home in the Jewish way of communicating with God.
6 x 9, 208 pp, Quality PB, 978-1-58023-201-2 **$18.99**

The Way Into Jewish Prayer Teacher's Guide
By Rabbi Jennifer Ossakow Goldsmith
8½ x 11, 42 pp, PB, 978-1-58023-345-3 **$8.99**
Download a free copy at www.jewishlights.com.

The Way Into Judaism and the Environment
By Jeremy Benstein, PhD
Explores the ways in which Judaism contributes to contemporary social-environmental issues, the extent to which Judaism is part of the problem and how it can be part of the solution.
6 x 9, 288 pp, Quality PB, 978-1-58023-368-2 **$18.99**; HC, 978-1-58023-268-5 **$24.99**

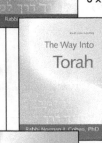

The Way Into Tikkun Olam (Repairing the World)
By Rabbi Elliot N. Dorff, PhD
An accessible introduction to the Jewish concept of the individual's responsibility to care for others and repair the world.
6 x 9, 304 pp, Quality PB, 978-1-58023-328-6 **$18.99**

The Way Into Torah
By Rabbi Norman J. Cohen, PhD
Helps guide you in the exploration of the origins and development of Torah, explains why it should be studied and how to do it.
6 x 9, 176 pp, Quality PB, 978-1-58023-198-5 **$16.99**

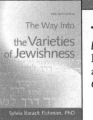

The Way Into the Varieties of Jewishness
By Sylvia Barack Fishman, PhD
Explores the religious and historical understanding of what it has meant to be Jewish from ancient times to the present controversy over "Who is a Jew?"
6 x 9, 288 pp, Quality PB, 978-1-58023-367-5 **$18.99**; HC, 978-1-58023-030-8 **$24.99**

Theology/Philosophy

From Defender to Critic: The Search for a New Jewish Self
By Dr. David Hartman
A daring self-examination of Hartman's goals, which were not to strip halakha of its authority but to create a space for questioning and critique that allows for the traditionally religious Jew to act out a moral life in tune with modern experience.
6 x 9, 336 pp, HC, 978-1-58023-515-0 **$35.00**

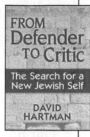

Our Religious Brains: What Cognitive Science Reveals about Belief, Morality, Community and Our Relationship with God
By Rabbi Ralph D. Mecklenburger; Foreword by Dr. Howard Kelfer; Preface by Dr. Neil Gillman
This is a groundbreaking, accessible look at the implications of cognitive science for religion and theology, intended for laypeople.   6 x 9, 224 pp, HC, 978-1-58023-508-2 **$24.99**

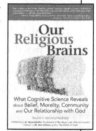

The Other Talmud—*The Yerushalmi*: Unlocking the Secrets of The Talmud of Israel for Judaism Today   *By Rabbi Judith Z. Abrams, PhD*
A fascinating—and stimulating—look at "the other Talmud" and the possibilities for Jewish life reflected there.   6 x 9, 256 pp, HC, 978-1-58023-463-4 **$24.99**

The Way of Man: According to Hasidic Teaching
By Martin Buber; New Translation and Introduction by Rabbi Bernard H. Mehlman and Dr. Gabriel E. Padawer; Foreword by Paul Mendes-Flohr
An accessible and engaging new translation of Buber's classic work—available as an e-book only.   E-book, 978-1-58023-601-0 Digital List Price **$14.99**

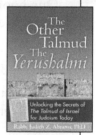

The Death of Death: Resurrection and Immortality in Jewish Thought
By Rabbi Neil Gillman, PhD   6 x 9, 336 pp, Quality PB, 978-1-58023-081-0 **$18.95**

Doing Jewish Theology: God, Torah & Israel in Modern Judaism *By Rabbi Neil Gillman, PhD*
6 x 9, 304 pp, Quality PB, 978-1-58023-439-9 **$18.99**; HC, 978-1-58023-322-4 **$24.99**

A Heart of Many Rooms: Celebrating the Many Voices within Judaism
By Dr. David Hartman   6 x 9, 352 pp, Quality PB, 978-1-58023-156-5 **$19.95**

The God Who Hates Lies: Confronting & Rethinking Jewish Tradition
By Dr. David Hartman with Charlie Buckholtz   6 x 9, 208 pp, HC, 978-1-58023-455-9 **$24.99**

Jewish Theology in Our Time: A New Generation Explores the Foundations and Future of Jewish Belief   *Edited by Rabbi Elliot J. Cosgrove, PhD; Foreword by Rabbi David J. Wolpe; Preface by Rabbi Carole B. Balin, PhD*   6 x 9, 240 pp, HC, 978-1-58023-413-9 **$24.99**

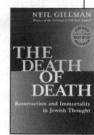

Maimonides—Essential Teachings on Jewish Faith & Ethics: The Book of Knowledge & the Thirteen Principles of Faith—Annotated & Explained
Translation and Annotation by Rabbi Marc D. Angel, PhD
5½ x 8½, 224 pp, Quality PB Original, 978-1-59473-311-6 **$18.99***

Maimonides, Spinoza and Us: Toward an Intellectually Vibrant Judaism
By Rabbi Marc D. Angel, PhD   6 x 9, 224 pp, HC, 978-1-58023-411-5 **$24.99**

A Touch of the Sacred: A Theologian's Informal Guide to Jewish Belief
By Dr. Eugene B. Borowitz and Frances W. Schwartz
6 x 9, 256 pp, Quality PB, 978-1-58023-416-0 **$16.99**; HC, 978-1-58023-337-8 **$21.99**

Traces of God: Seeing God in Torah, History and Everyday Life *By Rabbi Neil Gillman, PhD*
6 x 9, 240 pp, Quality PB, 978-1-58023-369-9 **$16.99**

Your Word Is Fire: The Hasidic Masters on Contemplative Prayer
Edited and translated by Rabbi Arthur Green, PhD, and Barry W. Holtz
6 x 9, 160 pp, Quality PB, 978-1-879045-25-5 **$15.95**

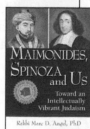

I Am Jewish
Personal Reflections Inspired by the Last Words of Daniel Pearl
Almost 150 Jews—both famous and not—from all walks of life, from all around the world, write about many aspects of their Judaism.
Edited by Judea and Ruth Pearl   6 x 9, 304 pp, Deluxe PB w/ flaps, 978-1-58023-259-3 **$18.99**
Download a free copy of the *I Am Jewish Teacher's Guide* at www.jewishlights.com.

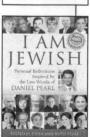

Hannah Senesh: Her Life and Diary, The First Complete Edition
By Hannah Senesh; Foreword by Marge Piercy; Preface by Eitan Senesh; Afterword by Roberta Grossman
6 x 9, 368 pp, b/w photos, Quality PB, 978-1-58023-342-2 **$19.99**

**A book from SkyLight Paths, Jewish Lights' sister imprint*

About Jewish Lights

People of all faiths and backgrounds yearn for books that attract, engage, educate, and spiritually inspire.

Our principal goal is to stimulate thought and help all people learn about who the Jewish People are, where they come from, and what the future can be made to hold. While people of our diverse Jewish heritage are the primary audience, our books speak to people in the Christian world as well and will broaden their understanding of Judaism and the roots of their own faith.

We bring to you authors who are at the forefront of spiritual thought and experience. While each has something different to say, they all say it in a voice that you can hear.

Our books are designed to welcome you and then to engage, stimulate, and inspire. We judge our success not only by whether or not our books are beautiful and commercially successful, but by whether or not they make a difference in your life.

For your information and convenience, at the back of this book we have provided a list of other Jewish Lights books you might find interesting and useful. They cover all the categories of your life:

Bar/Bat Mitzvah	Life Cycle
Bible Study / Midrash	Meditation
Children's Books	Men's Interest
Congregation Resources	Parenting
Current Events / History	Prayer / Ritual / Sacred Practice
Ecology / Environment	Social Justice
Fiction: Mystery, Science Fiction	Spirituality
Grief / Healing	Theology / Philosophy
Holidays / Holy Days	Travel
Inspiration	Twelve Steps
Kabbalah / Mysticism / Enneagram	Women's Interest

Stuart M. Matlins, Publisher

Or phone, fax, mail or e-mail to: **JEWISH LIGHTS Publishing**
Sunset Farm Offices, Route 4 • P.O. Box 237 • Woodstock, Vermont 05091
Tel: (802) 457-4000 • Fax: (802) 457-4004 • www.jewishlights.com
Credit card orders: (800) 962-4544 (8:30AM–5:30PM EST Monday–Friday)
Generous discounts on quantity orders. SATISFACTION GUARANTEED. Prices subject to change.

**For more information about each book,
visit our website at www.jewishlights.com**

✂ Cut along dotted lines and remove, fold as shown at center, tape closed and mail to Jewish Lights Publishing.

WIN A
$100
GIFT
CERTIFICATE!

Fill in this card and
mail it to us—
or fill it in online at

**jewishlights.com/
feedback.html**

—to be eligible for a
$100 gift certificate for
Jewish Lights books.

**JEWISH LIGHTS PUBLISHING
SUNSET FARM OFFICES RTE 4
PO BOX 237
WOODSTOCK VT 05091-0237**

Illumulullllumlumullllumulullulllumulullllumlullll

(fold here)

**Fill in this card and return it to us to be eligible for our
quarterly drawing for a $100 gift certificate for Jewish Lights books.**

We hope that you will enjoy this book and find it useful in enriching your life.

Book title: _____

Your comments: _____

How you learned of this book: _____

If purchased: Bookseller _____ City _____ State _____

Please send me a free JEWISH LIGHTS Publishing catalog. I am interested in: (check all that apply)

1. ❏ Spirituality
2. ❏ Mysticism/Kabbalah
3. ❏ Philosophy/Theology
4. ❏ History/Politics

5. ❏ Women's Interest
6. ❏ Environmental Interest
7. ❏ Healing/Recovery
8. ❏ Children's Books

9. ❏ Caregiving/Grieving
10. ❏ Ideas for Book Groups
11. ❏ Religious Education Resources
12. ❏ Interfaith Resources

Name (PRINT)_____

Street_____

City_____State_____Zip_____

E-MAIL (FOR SPECIAL OFFERS ONLY) _____

Please send a JEWISH LIGHTS Publishing catalog to my friend:

Name (PRINT) _____

Street _____

City_____State_____Zip_____

JEWISH LIGHTS PUBLISHING
Tel: (802) 457-4000 • Fax: (802) 457-4004
Available at better booksellers. Visit us online at www.jewishlights.com

Place
Stamp
Here